Autophagy

The Complete Guide to Build Your Body Balance With Intermittent Fasting Resistance Training, Grow Your Muscles, and Promote Longevity

By

Julie Water

☐ Copyright 2019 by ____Julie Water_____ - All rights reserved.

This content is provided with the sole purpose of providing relevant information on a specific topic for which every reasonable effort has been made to ensure that it is both accurate and reasonable. Nevertheless, by purchasing this content, you consent to the fact that the author, as well as the publisher, are in no way experts on the topics contained herein, regardless of any claims as such that may be made within. As such, any suggestions or recommendations that are made within are done so purely for entertainment value. It is recommended that you always consult a professional prior to undertaking any of the advice or techniques discussed within.

This is a legally binding declaration that is considered both valid and fair by both the Committee of Publishers Association and the American Bar Association and should be considered as legally binding within the United States.

The reproduction, transmission, and duplication of any of the content found herein, including any specific or extended information will be done as an illegal act regardless of the end form the information ultimately takes. This includes copied versions of the work both physical, digital and audio unless express consent of the Publisher is provided beforehand. Any additional rights reserved.

Furthermore, the information that can be found within the pages described forthwith shall be considered both accurate and truthful when it comes to the recounting of facts. As such, any use, correct or incorrect, of the provided information will render the Publisher free of responsibility as to the actions taken outside of their direct purview. Regardless, there are zero scenarios where the original author or the Publisher can be deemed liable in any fashion for any damages or hardships that may result from any of the information discussed herein.

Additionally, the information in the following pages is intended only for informational purposes and should thus be thought of as universal. As befitting its nature, it is presented without assurance regarding its prolonged validity or interim quality. Trademarks that are mentioned are done without written consent and can in no way be considered an endorsement from the trademark holder.

Table of Contents

Table of Contents

Chapter 1: Metabolic Autophagy in Terms of Diet and How It Works in Our Body

Chapter 2: Intermittent Fasting Diet and How It Relates to Metabolic Autophagy

Chapter 3: Metabolic Autophagy Hypertrophic Growth

Chapter 4: Anabolic Foods and Their Role

   One-Day Menu

   Sample Weekend Menu

   Low-Carb Meal Plan

   Sample Menu for High-Carb Diet

Chapter 5: Catabolic Foods and Their Role

   Catabolic Diet Meals

     Day One

     Day Two

     Day Three

     Day Four

     Day Five

     Day Six

     Day Seven

Chapter 6: Protein Absorption During Metabolic Autophagy
Chapter 7: How to Do Fasting
Chapter 8: When You Shouldn't Fast
Chapter 9: Types of Meals You Should Consume
Chapter 10: Metabolic Autophagy in Terms of Biology and Science
Chapter 11: Metabolic Autophagy While Sleeping
Chapter 12: Supplementation and Integration
Conclusion

Chapter 1: Metabolic Autophagy in Terms of Diet and How It Works in Our Body

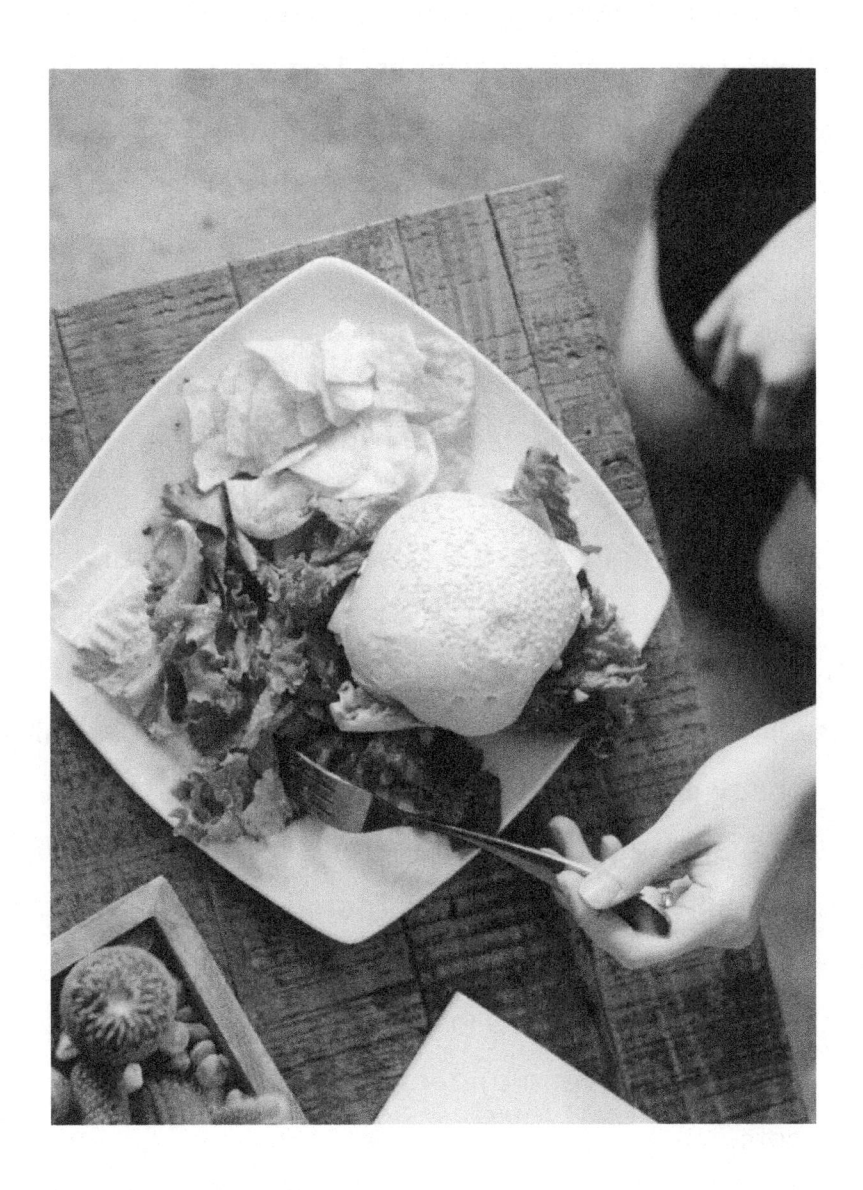

Autophagy is what is known as *cannibalization* but intended for your body. When your cells capture their own organelles along with their cytoplasm, they will consume them in the lysosomes. This results in a breakdown product. The products are inputs to metabolism that is cellular. Through this process of cellular metabolism, the inputs are used to generate energy, and they build new membranes and proteins.

The process of autophagy preserves the health of your tissues and cells by replacing cellular components that have been damaged or are outdated with fresh ones. An example that might make this easier to understand is to think of starvation. During this time, autophagy will provide you with a source of nutrients that's internal. This will offer energy generation and, in turn, survival. Autophagy can prevent degenerative diseases, and it acts as a strong promoter of metabolic homeostasis. All of this sounds amazing, right? There is a downside, however. Cancer cells love exploiting it and using it against you. Cancer cells love autophagy because they can use it to survive in tumors that are poor in nutrients.

Autophagy occurs at a low level constitutively. This is important to have quality control of intracellular through the constitutive turnover of the cytoplasmic component process. Autophagy pathways can be potently induced by things, such as the following:

- Hypoxia
- The stress of the oxidative kind
- An infection of the pathogen kind
- Exercise (physical)

It can also come from more serious things, such as nutrient deprivation or factors of growth. Their resulting macromolecules could be released and then become recycled back to what is known as the cytosol for a new biosynthesis process and production of energy. This helps to maintain the function of the cells under unfavorable conditions and survival under the same conditions.

This is different from other systems because other systems degrade primarily short-lived proteins, but autophagy is more than just self-destructive. It plays a role in a broader spectrum of physiological processes, which include some of the following examples.

- Cellular metabolism

- Energy homeostasis
- Development

There are three major types of autophagy, but we are going to be focusing on metabolic autophagy as our primary. In recent studies, it has been shown that autophagic machinery has defects. Those defects are associated with many different metabolic tissues like the following:

- Liver
- Adipose tissue
- Pancreatic B cells

It is also implicated in disorders of metabolism. They include the resistance of insulin and obesity. Unfortunately, autophagy can be implicated in metabolic diseases as well. Another issue with autophagy is that the transcriptional regulation of the machinery in organs is still unclear. Along with this, the roles of many additional factors of transcription and other factors in autophagy are still waiting to be discovered.

Autophagy is considered to be crucial for cellular metabolism maintenance when your experiencing nutrient deprivation. It is also involved in lipid metabolism. Autophagy is considered to be vital for functions of your neuronal, and as such, it exerts opposite effects on regulation of your metabolism in functionally antagonizing cell types of your neuronal. An example of this would be appetite-promoting neurons. These are known as an agouti-related peptide.

Studies have shown that at the cellular level, benefits can include these examples.

- Recycling of residual proteins
- Providing energy and being able to create building blocks for cells that are still able to benefit from repair
- Healthy cells and regeneration (however, this is on a larger scale, and that is worth noting)
- Removing toxic proteins that are from the cells that are attributed to neurodegenerative disease.

Autophagy also affects our diet as well. The two ways that you can trigger autophagy the quickest is through intermittent fasting and the ketogenic diet. Fasting has been said to be the most effective way to trigger autophagy in your body. The ketogenic diet helps as well because it puts your body into ketosis. The ketogenic diet is a diet where it takes fat as a major contributor. This diet is high in fat and low in carbs, but it brings the same benefits of fasting without actually having to fast.

Because of this, it's like a shortcut to induce the same beneficial metabolic changes. It is said that by not overwhelming the body with an external load, it gives the body a break to focus on its own health and repair. The keto diet offers you a very simple ratio of how you will get what you need. You get about 75% of your daily calories from fat, 20% of your calories from protein, and 5% from carbs. This sounds like a good idea and a safe diet, right? Unfortunately, we are wrong.

The problem with this diet is that doctors say that you shouldn't be on it for two major reasons—it can be fatal in certain cases and it puts your body into a state where your body is not meant to stay in. The ketogenic diet is mostly recommended for patients who are in extreme situations, and highly respected doctors say that you should only be on this diet for a matter of six months at most and never without the care or the watch of your doctor. In every situation with the diet, doctors say that you need constant care and to be in constant contact with health professionals because the diet simply isn't safe. So it's very important that you speak to a doctor before you even attempt the ketogenic diet.

There is a non-dieting way where you can activate autophagy. This is in the form of exercise. Now, this study needs more research on humans to be utterly conclusive, but studies performed on animals have proven that physical exercise can induce autophagy in organs that are part of your metabolic regulation process. However, there are more studies that need to be done. Nutritional and health experts point to the fact that there is still a lot we need to learn about autophagy and how best to encourage it for safety. If you are interested in stimulating autophagy in your body, however, it is recommended that you start exercising regularly and that you begin fasting, which is something that we're going to be talking about more. But first, you have to contact your doctor who can give you concrete advice and determine what is safe or unsafe for your body.

Intermittent fasting is another area that needs more study, in the same way that autophagy needs more research to be conclusive. It is said that intermittent fasting, as well as losing weight, can help you with autophagy, which is another reason that most people wish to attempt this. However, it has not been proven to be 100% safe, and fatalities have occurred from this as well.

There are different variations of this type of fasting, and studies have shown that they may be able to show you some good health benefits. Other reviews of the research conducted concluded that it may have positive effects, ranging from healthier body weight and lower risk of diseases to an increased lifespan. However, you should keep in mind that fasting is not recommended at all for children, people who have diabetes, and pregnant women. It's also not recommended unless your doctor gives you explicit instructions; as we have said before, it is not been proven to be 100% safe, and you shouldn't engage in things that can hurt you.

Exercising can put you in that state as well because working out damages your muscles, causing microscopic tears that your body rushes to 'fix.' This causes your muscles to become stronger and more resistant to any damage that you might cause them. Regular exercise is the most popular way to help our bodies cleanse themselves unintentionally. It is a healthy activity to engage in and has been said to help the body greatly. A study from a dozen years ago looked at the structures that form around the pieces of cells that the body has decided to recycle.

This study was done on mice, and they found that they were demolishing their own cells drastically and that it increased after they ran for a half an hour on a treadmill. As a note, however, it is hard to figure out the amount of exercise required to switch on this boost in humans. This is because there haven't been any conclusive studies in humans, so this needs more studying to actually be definite and conclusive. However, people are always looking for ways to induce autophagy through chemicals because it would be easier than dieting, but there are two wrong things with this desire. The first is that chemicals are dangerous to the human body and could be fatal, and second, we're a long way from this because we haven't been able to prove that it's safe. Obviously, safety is the most important thing with whatever you do.

There are many metabolic changes that take place in different areas of your life and body. There are patterns that you might use for yourself. However, the ketogenic diet and staying in the state of ketosis is not recommended because of the bodily stress that comes with it and the fact that it can be fatal.

It's also an important note to remember that you don't have to exercise or fast all day to receive these benefits. In fact, doing so will harm you in ways that you can't foresee. Even a few hours here and there can help, but as we've said before, you need to talk to your doctor first to make sure that you're doing the best thing for your body. The same is true for exercise; everyone is different and needs different things. As such, you need to have the guidance of health professionals before attempting anything because you could end up hurting yourself beyond repair.

Another effect of autophagy that might be able to help you understand what it is and why it's so important is the cellular damage it's supposed to fix and the issues that can occur if not handled properly. We incur cellular damage every day, and part of it occurs from things that we just happen to walk into. Examples include pollution, solar radiation, viruses from other people, or infectious bacteria, but other forms of damage are simple and a byproduct of how we live.

Metabolism creates invaders that can damage your DNA, and while your adaptive immune system creates an instrument to deal with these invaders, the immune system is supposed to act as a tool that will quickly smash what is attacking you and all the surrounding tissue before they can take hold inside you.

The system that creates chemicals like hypochlorite or hydrogen peroxide to handle the attackers can be activated to help your body get rid of what's not supposed to be there. Autophagy is meant to be a quick response that is vital for survival, but it can cause damage to your cells that you didn't intend to cause at the same time.

If a cell obtains DNA damage, it loses the skill to divide, and it becomes senescent. This isn't what we want because they can have too much damage and cause harm if they keep doing this. This is a vital healing process and defense mechanism for your body to help deal with stress. If a cell that has DNA damage divides, then it could make a dangerous mutation spread in your system, and this can become carcinogenic, which is obviously dangerous.

When a cell becomes senescent, it does a few different things. Some of them include the fact that it stops replicating, where it sends signaling molecules to tell your body that the hurt cell should be replaced and destroyed.

Autophagy is supposed to occur mainly in the absence of food, which is why intermittent fasting is believed to be the best trigger for it. We live in a world where calorie-heavy foods are constantly available to us. Since this is the case, most people hardly ever, if ever at all, activate this system. This would cause the damaged or senescent cells in your body to accumulate. As they stack up, they're going to pump out inflammatory signals that encourage your system to supply a steady dose of that hydrogen peroxide to all of the surrounding cells. This is going to cause them to incur constant damage, thereby aging far more rapidly than they do now.

In addition to these growth factors that were supposed to help their replacement cell, they're going to push the damaged cell over the edge to become a cancerous cell. So many people see chronic inflammation as the cause of aging in general. More to the point, chronic inflammation causes poor aging, and it makes all of the surrounding cells function poorly and age far more rapidly than they're supposed to. Even things like graying hair or thinning hair are caused by senescent cells that harm their neighboring hair follicles, turning them weaker. As such, the senescent cells also trigger decreased function in our immune system. This focuses us on relying more on the innate immune system. As we get older, your body relies more and more on that tool to hammer away what's not supposed to be there.

Autophagy is also supposed to restore proper function, and recent research is pointing out how vital it is to successful aging. However, since the research has only been done on mice, and mice are different from us, we need more conclusive answers and studies.

Immune function is something that does normally decreases as we age and as the adaptive immune system declines. Autophagy is supposed to restore this adaptive immune function and prevent the switch that is related to age to increase the activation system. Instead, this grants us a greater response to infection, along with being able to help keep your inflammation in check. This is why many people try fasting in the first place. They want to activate this for their body and their health. They are also interested in the fact that autophagy is supposed to prevent diseases and slow down the aging process.

A lot of things about autophagy are still too early to be proven to be definitive. Though it is believed to help you in a beneficial way, there is one fundamental problem with this reasoning. Studies have shown that it is very difficult to monitor in a living organism, especially a human.

Until we can study humans more efficiently, we can't prove that autophagy is completely safe. There is also too much debate regarding its effect on cancer, as well as other areas. This just shows that we need better research and studies on autophagy for the future.

Chapter 2: Intermittent Fasting Diet and How It Relates to Metabolic Autophagy

Intermittent fasting has been studied in relation to autophagy and is believed to kick the process off. Studies believe that fasting is how we can get our bodies into an autophagic state. It is believed that autophagy is an advanced form of fasting, so there is now a new interest in both subjects and as to how they really relate to each other, functioning together or apart. Autophagy is now going mainstream because fasting is going mainstream as well. More people want to know about these topics because they believe it could be the key to losing weight. However, as we have said in other chapters, fasting and autophagy have not been proven to be entirely safe, and they still need more research.

The key difference between autophagy and intermittent fasting is the way people use them. People who want to fast believe that they would lose weight with it. Also, fasting allows them to control or maintain weight loss. While those who attempt to trigger autophagy do so to protect them against certain diseases, using the self-cannibalism process of autophagy.

We've already discussed the basic idea behind autophagy and how it relates to food, as well as its effectiveness against certain diseases like cancer and dementia, among others. However, as mentioned before, it still needs conclusive studies.

Autophagy is induced in a wide variety of organs in response to food deprivation, and more studies are being conducted to give the best information possible so that we can know the benefits of both. Some experts have suspected that fasting needs to last twenty-four hours or longer to be able to trigger autophagy; however, this is not clear. This is because the twenty-four-hour test was done on mice, and the metabolism of mice doesn't necessarily correspond to the metabolism of a human.

There have been interviews conducted with nephrologists (kidney doctor), and there have been interviews conducted with fasting researchers. They have suggested that at possibly around twenty to twenty-four hours is where your autophagy would be activated, but this is an educated guess and has no conclusive proof.

Researchers have a special interest in the way autophagy and fasting-induced autophagy, in particular, interacts with cancer, although the effects are unclear and very complicated. This is partly due to the fact that cancer is confused and weakened by fasting, and if you take traditional medicine, such as chemotherapy (which is what many cancer patients have to take), then research has shown that autophagy is not necessarily safe unless you get permission from your doctor. Other studies have shown that autophagy can have the exact opposite effect, which makes tumors stronger and more resistant to radiation, which can keep you sick longer because the medicine is not working the way that it needs to. Autophagy is said to play a dual role in cancer because it acts as both a suppressor to the tumors and a mechanism to promote the growth of tumors. Because of this, autophagy and fasting are very controversial. There is a debate on whether or not autophagy manipulation should be attempted at all in cancer therapy, and the same is true of fasting. There are also concerns that fasting-induced weight loss and too much of it could be dangerous, especially among cancer patients.

No study on fasting-induced autophagy has been conducted on people yet, so the information we have, though good, is not entirely conclusive. There were papers published regarding autophagy, but there are holes in the research that need to be filled with an actual study on humans, which is currently in the works. Autophagy is seen as a double-edged sword because of its ability to mitigate injuries or exacerbate them, as we have mentioned earlier. At the same time, fasting has also been shown to contribute to the development of gallstones. In addition, intermittent fasting and autophagy could overlap with anorexia. It is also said that when it comes to metabolic autophagy, fasting should only be attempted by a healthy person twice a year and no more.

It is believed that when you fast, you are doing it for the greater good of your body. What this means is that when you are fasting, you do it because you believe that it's going to help your body in some way, such as losing weight, influencing the outcome of a medical issue, or preventing a certain medical issue from taking place. For years, researchers have been eager to understand why fasting is linked to autophagy and longevity, but they have only tested it on lab mice. In these tests, the mice were brought in a state of fasting, and they were observed if they would live longer than their peers that are fed regularly. They're also trying to see their autophagic structures to compare them.

Human research has been able to find that restricting calories turns on genes that tell cells to preserve resources. When this happens, the cells go into a preservation mode. This is also known as famine mode. In this mode, your cells are believed to be much more resistant to cellular stress or disease. They will also enter a process known to us as autophagy, which is what we are trying to understand. These particular studies may have only been able to test mice, but scientists are hopeful of having better information within the next few years.

We have to be careful with what we know about the autophagy studies because it is difficult to measure outside of a lab environment. Studies suggest that the process in humans may initiate only after eighteen hours of fasting, and the maximum benefits occur once the forty-eight-hour mark has been reached, but more studies need to be done to be sure. For many people, this amount of time (forty-eight hours) sounds daunting and complicated as well, but for those who have their doctor's permission to do this, it is believed that fasts are supposed to give you your desired benefits. Remember, however, that you're only supposed to do this periodically, as it puts too much strain on your body.

Attempting to stimulate this through intermittent fasting is believed to help the production of your growth hormones and regenerate our cellular material in your body. It is also believed that if your body has recently had an infection, it may be able to destroy lingering bacteria or viruses once you enter the autophagy mode.

Also, when autophagy does not take place frequently, and the body collects a variety of different cellular material, proteins in the body can build up. Researchers believe that prolonged bouts of autophagy may be able to help clear out the brain of excess proteins that are noted to be in patients with cancer and other unfortunate diseases like Parkinson's.

In preclinical studies, a dietary restriction was shown to extend lifespan and reduce the development of diseases related to age. These include diseases, such as cancer, diabetes, and even cardiovascular diseases. The dietary restrictions promoted metabolic and cellular changes in organisms that allow periods of limited nutrient availability. The main changes that they found include decreased blood glucose levels, growth factor signaling, and the activation of resistance of stress pathways, which affected the cell growth, among other issues.

Nutrient starvation, as we have already said, is going to activate your autophagy, but other studies were able to demonstrate that if you have a dietary intervention, it may also reduce tumor incidents and other issues. As everyone wants to be as healthy as they can, this may be a helpful way to begin. Fasting is still undergoing intense investigation relating to oncology, and it has yielded interesting results, which makes us excited for more solid information in the future. Fasting is characterized by the complete deprivation of food (in some cases, as there are many different forms of fasting) but not water.

Other fasting methods, such as intermittent fasting, allows you to eat, so there are different studies conducted on both to see which would be more useful. There have been intermittent fasting protocols being performed because we can deduce that science and research are both interested in knowing if intermittent fasting can help cancer treatments in humans, as well as in animals.

Intermittent fasting, as shown in a study with mice, showed that by reducing the circulating glucose levels, the mice were then protected from certain toxicity, and they were promoted in protection as well. As of today, there are other clinical trials involving intermittent fasting combined with chemotherapy in cancer patients so that in the future, we will see how effective it is. The result of these trials will be vital for a better evaluation of clinical potential and the application of a new therapeutic strategy that would involve fasting.

Diet had been shown as a modulator for health in the kidneys in humans and experimental models that science is looking into. As we speak, calorie restriction is being studied, and the effects of doing so have shown that it may possibly slow down the associated molecular physiological or even pathological processes from progressing. These can occur in tissues with high oxidative demand, for example, in kidneys, heart, or brain. In contrast, when they fed the mice with a high-calorie diet, the mice became obese. They had cardiovascular diseases and other issues, including metabolic disorders and a shortened lifespan. This is where autophagy comes in. Autophagy is self-cannibalizing, which means that it's supposed to be feeding off you when you are in fasting mode, as this is critical for survival. During nutrient deprivation, this is where the fasting in the autophagy is linked because they are supposed to help you regenerate or renew your cells. It is also believed that fasting is much better than a high-calorie diet because a high-calorie diet can cause so much damage to your body.

Eating a high-calorie diet, not exercising, or eating calories of the wrong kind, such as cheeseburgers is going to cause damage to your body. In this case, people believe fasting would be the better choice when they should really be focusing on eating the right foods.

Because autophagy prevents many things, you can use intermittent fasting as a way to help; fasting triggers autophagy in the first place.

With that said, you could use both fasting and autophagy to your advantage.

Chapter 3: Metabolic Autophagy Hypertrophic Growth

Hypertrophy, or nourishment, is the increase in the volume of an organ or tissue caused by the enlargement of its component cells. It is distinguished from hyperplasia. Hyperplasia and hypertrophic growth are two different processes, and they are distinct, but they frequently occur together, such as in cases of hormone-induced proliferation and enlargement of the cells and the uterus during pregnancy.

There are different types of hypertrophy, and hypertrophic growth can occur in many different ways. It can occur in cardiac myocytes, as well as different functions of the body. In this chapter, we're going to specifically be looking at hypertrophic growth and how it relates to autophagy.

Cells have a very interesting drive to enlarge their mass, and that's illustrated in the growth of embryos and juveniles during development. However, even in all organisms which have already reached a steady-state, they continue to grow. If differentiated stems and stem cells allow for the replacement of damaged cells, the process of cell growth has a humongous energetic need, and it's rapidly abandoned if conditions become unfavorable. The coupling of autophagy and growth might appear to be intuitive and logical, but the potential cause-and-effect relationships between the two, as well as the underlying mechanisms that link them are beginning to be unraveled. If you're able to understand the psychological benefits of this coordination and the consequences of its disruption, you should be able to have a better insight into autophagy.

Autophagy is also believed to modulate hypertrophy in the heart and the setting of hemodynamic stress. An example would be something like hypertension. The heart will undergo a compensatory hypertrophic growth response. This hypertrophic response triggers a myocyte death and a clinical syndrome of heart failure. For years, autophagy has been implanted in the pathophysiology of heart failure. On the other hand, a potent activator of autophagy prevents cardiac hypertrophy induced by thyroid hormone treatment. This treatment and can even regress established cardiac hypertrophy that is induced by pressure overload and improve your cardiac function. Because of this, it is believed that autophagy might be able to work with hypertrophic growth, and it might also antagonize cardiac hypertrophy by increasing protein degradation, which would decrease cardiac mass.

Hypertrophy and hypertrophic growth also occur in muscles. Muscle hypertrophy is a term for the growth and increase of muscle cells, and the most common type of this occurs as a result of physical exercise. When you start exercising a muscle, there is an increase in the nerve that will cause muscle contraction.

This can often result in strength gains without any noticeable change in actual muscle size. As you continue to exercise, there will be a complex interaction of nervous system responses that result in an increase in protein synthesis. Over the months that you are doing this, the muscle cells begin to grow larger and stronger. Although the process of hypertrophy is the same for everyone, your results are different from others doing the same workout. This is due to the difference in the genetic makeup of your muscles.

For some people, the process of hypertrophic growth occurs at a much larger degree or at a faster rate than it does in others. The appearance of a muscle and the shape of a muscle are additional factors that vary and are based on your genetics. In this case, hypertrophy and autophagy work together well because when you exercise, your autophagy will kick in stronger, and it will be able to help your body. Remember, as we have said before in previous chapters, intermittent fasting and exercise are both believed to trigger autophagy. However, when you are fasting, you need to keep your exercises to a minimum.

Hypertrophy is something that is not fully understood, and this is true, particularly in the exact signals that cause tissues to hypertrophy during periods of increased functional demands. Hormones and growth factors play a role in hypertrophic growth and in autophagy. Regardless of the mechanism, there is an increase in synthesis and enzymes so that the cell is able to keep up with the increase in demand and metabolic activity. Remember that hypertrophy is an increase in cell size, not the actual number of cells themselves. Weightlifting can result in larger muscles, but the increase in muscle size is not caused by an increase in cell number but to an increase in the number and size of the myofibrils.

Hypertrophy can also be a compensatory process as well. When an organ or a portion of an organ is failing or has already failed, the other organ or portion of the organ is called upon to do more work. Because of this, hypertrophy is activated to meet the increased demand. For example, if a kidney was atrophied, then the other kidney would become enlarged. Cellular hypertrophy can result from the proliferation of a specific organelle as well. That makes the function of oxidases in the endoplasmic reticulum of hepatocytes responsible for detoxifying a variety of drugs and chemicals.

The liver response to increased demand for detoxification by increased hepatocyte SER. This will result in hypertrophy of these hepatocytes. Hypertrophy is a prominent response to chronic administration. Cellular hypertrophy and cellular hyperplasia are common responses to stimuli.

Through exercise, your muscular work is being done against the progressively challenging overload, which, as we have mentioned, increases in muscle mass, which is referred to as hypertrophy, but even though intense research has been done on the subject, scientists still don't fully understand hypertrophy and how it relates to autophagy and other parts of your body. They also don't understand completely how the muscle adapts to gradually overloading stimuli. The physiology of muscle hypertrophy is explored, and the interaction of the satellite cells and immune system reactions are explored, as well. In many different studies, the satellite cells are supposed to function to facilitate the growth and maintenance of damaged skeletal muscle tissue but not cardiac muscle tissue, which may surprise you.

The cells are satellite cells because they are located on the outer surface of the fiber of your muscle. Usually, these cells are dormant, but once they have become activated, when your muscle receives any form of trauma or injury, the satellite cells then multiply, and they're drawn to the damaged muscle site. It's important to emphasize that the process is not creating more muscle fibers in humans but is actually increasing in size of the contractual proteins within the muscle fiber. The growth factors are highly specific proteins, which can include hormones involved in muscle hypertrophy. The growth factor stimulates the differentiation and the division of a particular type of cell concerning skeletal muscle hypertrophy and hypertrophic growth factors of particular interest. These include insulin-like growth. The growth factors work in conjunction with each other to cause what is known as hypertrophy of the skeletal muscle. As you can see, autophagy plays an important role in your body, and there's also another part that hypertrophic growth can play in both metabolic autophagy and your body. The link between the two stems from how they affect your muscles and the inner workings of your cells, particularly in the aspect of your muscles and their growth. It's important to understand how both of these affect your body because everyone wants to be healthy and understands their health as best as they can to reap its benefits. Understanding these aspects is going to help you see how they treat and affect your body in different ways and if they are safe to try and engage in. It's also beneficial to understand how they're used for your benefit, which is an important part of understanding your body and its inner workings and how you can get the inner workings to work for your health. Autophagy is a very interesting subject as is hypertrophy, so learning what we can is an important part of being informed.

Chapter 4: Anabolic Foods and Their Role

Anabolism is a type of metabolism process where the chemical reaction leads to the synthesis of molecules or atoms to form larger molecules. The other type of metabolism is catabolism, which works in contrast to anabolism. Here, the molecules are broken down. These processes are called metabolic pathways, which comprise a series of chemical reactions happening inside a cell. Another difference between these two is that the anabolic process utilizes energy, while the catabolic process releases it.

Since anabolism forms large molecules, catabolism breaks them down. Energy is used to build chemical bonds between the nutrient molecules or 'macromolecules' in an anabolic process. These macromolecules are utilized when repairing the cell or building new ones. These metabolic processes are governed by our circadian rhythms, and they are crucial to the development, growth, and repair or maintenance of the cell. Certain hormones, anabolic in nature, activate your anabolic pathways, and they facilitate cellular growth. Some examples of such chemicals are testosterone and insulin.

There are different examples of the anabolic process. The three most popular are DNA synthesis, protein synthesis, and the growth of your muscles and bones. Protein synthesis is a process that involves how proteins affect your body. Proteins or macromolecules can better accomplish cellular activities. This means is that they have a lot of different functions in your body. This includes DNA replication, helping your enzymes, chemical reactions, cell growth, and other similar processes.

Each cell in the human body houses billions of proteins. Amino acids are protein molecules that are synthesized together in the ribosomes of the cell. Each protein comprises a particular sequence of amino acids. This process where protein is synthesized is therefore anabolic in nature, in the same way that bone and muscle growth, as well as overall growth of the body, are all anabolic. The growth of the bone or ossification forms through osteoclasts, which are mineralized through osteoblasts that is responsible for the production of calcium phosphate crystals. These are incorporated in the bone structure, resulting in hard and sturdy bones. Another anabolic process, muscle growth, takes place when myocytes also grow. These are skeletal muscle cells, which are strengthened through the use of muscles, such as exercising or weight-lifting.

Now that you know what anabolism is and what it does, we can talk about the foods you can eat. The foods that can help you with this type of diet range from cheap to expensive, as with any other diet that you know. But you should remember you'll need to purchase natural and wholesome foods that are anabolic in order to utilize their effects. Whole eggs are going to be a big staple for you. The protein content is good; the saturated fat and the cholesterol are alright because eggs are loaded with happy cholesterol.

An important note, however, is that you will need to eat both the egg whites and yolk. If you just eat the egg whites and throw away the yolk, then you're depriving yourself of vital enhancing compounds, and it's going to spike your insulin, which is something that you don't need.

Kale is great as well if it's raw. The meat and potatoes that people talk about all the time are great protein, but you shouldn't forget the micronutrients that you need as well. Kale is good because it's full of vitamins; oats and Greek yogurt are great options as well, as long the oats are rolled and old-fashioned, and the Greek yogurt is plain. Another great option is coconut oil, provided that it is extra virgin and unrefined. The refined version is full of chemicals because the oil had been deodorized and bleached. This makes it full of trans fat that you should be avoiding.

You can use frozen blueberries, unsweetened, if they're the wild Maine version, which you can find in the frozen section, usually for a low price. These are a great source of micronutrients and can be added to literally to any dish or smoothie. The best part is that they are affordable in a way that fresh blueberries are not. Fresh fruit goes on sale much less than frozen ones.

Bananas are also a cheap food that is a great source of potassium. Many eat them after a workout. You can have potatoes of all types, especially sweet potatoes and red potatoes. Red potatoes are a very cost-effective way to get in some great nutrients, but sweet potatoes are great sources of vitamin A and other nutrients. Red potatoes do not carry vitamin A, but they do have magnesium.

Other foods that you can have on this diet are turkey burgers. This is a processed food, so it's not highly recommended, but they made the list because they are low in sodium and have a high protein content. The calories are low, but the fat is something to be aware of.

You can also have coffee, which is probably making you smile as you read this. Everyone loves coffee, and thankfully, coffee is fairly cheap, and it has an array of antioxidants if it's a nice medium roast.

Other foods that are good for anabolism are meats that include the following:

- red meats
- salami
- sausage
- pork
- beef

Poultry, including the following:

- turkey
- chicken

Fish or shellfish that include the following:

- lobster
- shrimp
- crab

You can also have dairy, which includes cheese and eggs, along with healthy fats like olive oil or butter. Along with this, you can have a variety of vegetables, including the following:

- spinach
- cucumbers
- asparagus
- celery

You're also allowed to have certain fruits, as long as they stay within what you need. You can have berries and watermelon because they have very few carbs, but if you eat too many of them, your daily total is going to go up to far.

You can also drain calorie-free flavored beverages. Just remember that you need to avoid hidden carbs that are not allowed with anabolic foods.

One-Day Menu

A sample one-day menu for an anabolic diet would be the following. Keep in mind that these meals are just for the anabolic diet.

Meal one:

- A single tablespoon of oil
- A single ounce of cheese. It needs to be cheddar
- Three eggs. Use whole eggs.
- A duo of turkey sausage links. Cooked.

You're going to cook the eggs and cheese in the oil after whisking the two together. Then cook your sausage.

Snack one:

- A single tablespoon of oil
- A single tablespoon of almond butter
- A single tablespoon of flaxseed meal
- Six ounces of cottage cheese. It needs to be one percent

Mix everything into your cottage cheese.

Meal two:

- One tablespoon of vinegar
- Chicken breast cooked and four ounces

- Romaine lettuce two cups
- A single egg. Hard-boiled.
- Two tablespoons of oil

Serve your ingredients over lettuce. Toss it with the vinegar and oil.

Snack two:

- Two tablespoons of peanut butter
- One ounce cheese. Make sure it's cheddar.
- Ground beef. Make it sure its four ounces.

Cook beef with cheese and serve peanut butter on the side.

Meal three:

- Half a tablespoon of vinegar
- One tablespoon of oil
- Chicken breast. Make sure it's cooked and four ounces.
- Romaine lettuce. You will need two cups.
- One tablespoon of flaxseed meal

Whisk the ingredients in a bowl (not including the lettuce and chicken). Toss with the lettuce and serve with the chicken.

Sample Weekend Menu

A sample weekend menu could be as follows. Remember that the portions are going to vary based on your individual calorie needs.

Meal one:

Omelet using egg white, fresh fruit, and pancakes

Meal two:

Chicken breast and pasta. Use tomato sauce and garlic bread

Meal three:

Turkey breast inside a bagel with low-fat cheese

Meal four:

A ground beef hamburger that is extra-lean and a sweet potato

Meal five:

Shrimp tacos that are served over beans and rice

Low-Carb Meal Plan

Another sample of a meal plan that would last for a day and is low carb would be the following.

Meal one:

- Four slices of bacon, cooked.
- Over easy eggs. You may have two.

Meal two:

- Two ounces of deli meat
- Three ounces of cheese

Meal three:

- Three ounces of cheese, string cheese
- Two ounces of pepperoni.

Meal four:

- A single tablespoon of mustard
- Turkey hotdogs. You may have two of them.

Meal five:

- One-half of a tablespoon of vinegar
- A single tablespoon of oil. Use olive oil.
- Carrots, either steamed or raw. You will need one cup.
- Turkey breast, ten ounces
- Romaine lettuce. You will need two cups.

Meal six:

- A single ounce of cheese
- A single ounce of nuts

Sample Menu for High-Carb Diet

A high-carb diet for anabolism is the following.

Meal one:

- Two tablespoons of jelly
- English muffin, whole wheat. You may have two of them.

Meal two:

- Half a dozen crackers, whole wheat
- A single cup of fruit salad

Meal three:

- One-half of a tablespoon of butter
- One and a half cups of cooked brown rice
- Whole wheat toast. You may enjoy two slices.
- Four ounces of chili with beans

Meal four:

A single bowl of cereal with a cup and a half of milk that is nonfat

Meal five:

- A single ounce of turkey
- One single teaspoon of mustard
- Two lettuce leaves, and two slices of tomatoes
- Two slices of bread. Whole wheat is needed.
- Two cups of drained canned yams
- A single tablespoon of mayonnaise that is fat-free

Meal six:

- Two tablespoons of jelly
- A single bagel. It needs to be whole wheat

Keep in mind that these meals will vary from person to person as their needs and health are different, but this should give you a basic idea of what an anabolic diet looks like.

Chapter 5: Catabolic Foods and Their Role

Catabolism is what happens when you digest food, and your molecules break down in the body for use as energy. This means that when you digest food, the molecules break down, and your body uses them as energy. Large complex molecules in the body are broken down into smaller, simpler ones. An example of catabolism is glycolysis. This is the process that is almost the exact reverse of gluconeogenesis. Understanding catabolism can help you understand what you need to do for your body and how you can get healthier, although you need a doctor's watchful eye to make sure that you're doing this correctly. The hormones that are involved in catabolism are the following:

- Adrenaline
- Cortisol
- Cytokines
- And many others as well

Catabolism is a set of biochemical reactions that break down the complex molecules in your body into simpler ones. The process that it makes is thermodynamically favorable and spontaneous. This means that your cells use them to generate energy or to be the fuel for anabolism. Catabolism is what is known as exogenic, which means that it releases heat, and it works via oxidation and hydrolysis.

Cells can be beneficial to you in that they are able to store useful raw material in the complex molecules, and they can use catabolism to break them down and recover the smaller molecules to build new products for your body. A great example is the catabolism of proteins. Sometimes, waste products are generated, including ammonia, acidic acid, carbon dioxide, and other serious things of that nature.

Catabolism processes are the reverse of the anabolic processes, and they used to generate energy for those anabolic processes that need energy. They also release small molecules for other purposes such as detoxifying chemicals and regulating your metabolic pathways. Many hormones work as a signal to control catabolism, and most catabolic exercises, such as a cardio workout or another type of aerobic exercise.

Catabolic foods are supposed to burn up more calories than they supply, and this is because they require your body to work hard to metabolize them. The basic idea here is that you're burning more than you're taking in. For instance, an apple has 85 calories (give or take; it depends on the size) in each one you eat. This is an example of catabolic food because it burns 99 calories. It is catabolic through the process of burning more than you're taking in. Our bodies are extremely complex, however, and this requires further study so that we have more concrete information. Food behaves in a different way in different bodies, and most are high in fiber, which is good for you, no matter what kind of calories you're taking in.

It is thought that this will help you maintain your weight, and it would be helpful to eat these types of foods each day. Even with these types of foods, you should also be eating others as well, including protein. They believe that you can eat carbs in moderation without gaining weight. This is as long as you're watching yourself and making sure you stay within certain levels.

High-grade catabolic foods are believed to be more effective than others when it comes to catabolism, and it's best to consume your foods over the course of an entire day and spread it out. It is very important, as shown in certain studies that you spread them out instead of doing them in a single sitting because this is better for your body and your health.

There are different high-grade catabolic foods that primarily include fruits and vegetables.

With fruits, you can eat things like the following:

- limes
- oranges
- blackberries
- blueberries
- pineapple
- plums
- cantaloupe
- pears
- strawberries
- lemons
- grapefruit
- raspberries, as long as they are fresh
- watermelon

You can also have vegetables, such as the following:

- asparagus

- broccoli
- parsley
- cucumbers
- peppers
- tomato
- radishes
- zucchini
- Brussel sprouts
- carrots
- celery
- eggplant
- cooked leeks
- spinach
- sweet potatoes

Then there are low-grade catabolic foods that you can eat, and they include those same sections.

You can eat seafood that includes the following:

- Tuna
- Crabs
- Flounder
- Cooked lobster
- Shrimp
- Cod

- Mussels

You can have fruit, such as the following:

- Peaches
- Cherries
- Apricots
- Peaches
- Tangerines
- Nectarines
- Melon (honeydew)
- Apples
- Grapes

The vegetables that will be good for you to eat are the following:

- Cabbage (red)
- Beets
- Cauliflower
- Corn
- Green beans
- String beans
- chives
- Garlic
- Onions
- Peas

- Pumpkin
- Turnips
- Dill pickles

A sample meal plan for seven days on a catabolic diet could look like the following. We will be splitting it into five parts—meal one, snack, meal two, snack, and dinner. Keep in mind that the meal plans are just for the catabolic diet.

Catabolic Diet Meals

Day One

Meal one:

Scrambled eggs with broccoli and spinach topped with butter

Snack one:

Roasted seaweed and almonds

Meal two:

Caesar salad (with no croutons) and baked chicken for the salad

Snack two:

A protein shake

Meal three:

Stir fry with onions, peppers, and bok choy with fried chicken breast

Day Two

Meal one:

A pair of eggs over easy with sea salt and butter

Snack one:

Yogurt. It needs to be Greek.

Meal two:

Baked chicken salad with beets and dressing. The dressing will need to be low-carb.

Snack two:

A protein shake

Meal three:

Chicken breast. You will need to bake it and serve with asparagus and butter.

Day Three

Meal one:

Omelet with onions and peppers. Top it with a half avocado with butter.

Snack one:

Yogurt. Make sure it's Greek.

Meal two:

Leftover salad from the day before.

Snack two:

A protein shake

Meal three:

Steamed broccoli and butter with three poached eggs

Day Four

Meal one:

Turkey sausage with over-easy eggs

Snack one:

Celery and peanut butter (almond butter)

Meal two:

Chicken and lettuce wraps with salsa

Snack two:

Protein shake

Meal three:

Sautéed bok choy with lamb chops (make sure they are grass-fed)

Day Five

Meal one:

Two sausage links and scrambled eggs with spinach.

Snack one:

Small apple with peanut butter (almond butter)

Meal two:

Leftover stir fry

Snack two:

Protein shake

Meal three:

Lettuce chicken wraps with salsa

Day Six

Meal one:

Eggs (hardboiled) with sea salt, and olive oil

Snack one:

Seaweed snack, roasted

Meal two:

Steamed broccoli and butter and a stuffed burger

Snack two:

Protein shake

Meal three:

Sautéed zucchini and broccoli with baked chicken breast. Use a tomato cream sauce.

Day Seven

Meal one:

Two sausage links and scrambled eggs with broccoli

Snack one:

Yogurt. Make sure it's Greek.

Meal two:

Side salad with a dressing that is low-carb, along with a stuffed burger

Snack two:

Protein shake

Meal three:

Sautéed Brussel sprouts and baked chicken breast

By eating these foods, you should be able to activate the catabolic process that you are trying to achieve. Catabolic foods are very similar to negative calorie foods, and many of the basic principles are shared with both of them. The main idea that both of them share is that certain foods require more calories during the digestion process than they provide. This means that when they're consumed, they encourage your body to call on its fat stores and energy reserves. It has been said that you will lose weight faster with such foods.

Promoters of these claims tell people that they will lose weight faster by eating these foods than any other way. They encourage eating healthy foods over unhealthy foods or dangerous behavior. While the wording of their claims seems pretty nice, there are still important things to take in. They claim that if you eat these foods, your body's digestion system works hard to burn the calories taken on board, and the body will burn more calories than it normally does, which will use up more energy that will be drawn out of the fat reserves. This is described as an inner body way to exercise, or in simpler terms, this is an exercise that your inner body is conducting.

The principles of this line of thinking are not new. People have been talking about this for a very long time, and it's been around since the last century. An interesting thing to note is that these ideas have actually decreased in popularity because of the restricted foods that can be eaten and because they share many of the same traits as other diets. Some catabolic foods have suggested combining these with low protein sources, and others claim that they can combat the calories contained within anything that you eat with it. However, many studies have shown that this isn't necessarily true, while others swear that it is. There has been much debate back and forth on just how much catabolic foods can do for us. On the subject of diet or following the ideas of catabolic food, they say they will help you with your health and mind, but there are a few things to remember when thinking about this. Studies have shown that this may not be entirely accurate, so you should talk to your doctor or a nutritionist. This is because they can give you the correct information that you need, and they will be able to tell you how much you can do for your body and how to do it safely.

If you want to ingest catabolic foods, then you need to eat the actual vegetables or fruit and don't consume them in juice form because those are full of sugar and excess things that you don't need in your system. You should also drink plenty of water as it's recommended for a healthy body, and you need to remember that your body can only handle so much water at once, so be careful not to overhydrate. Still, make sure that you are drinking enough water to stay hydrated and healthy.

Another thing to remember is to stop right away if you experience any unusual side effects or become uncomfortable because that's your body telling you that something is wrong. There are websites that make very wild and unsubstantiated claims by medical professionals about catabolic foods, and this is why you need to talk to your doctor before doing anything and to remember that if something sounds too good to be true, then it often is not true. You should never put your health at risk by following a certain line of thinking or claims.

The thing that you should remember is that there is no magic food that can help you lose weight, which is one of the big reasons that people want to explore catabolic foods in the first place. Instead, you should focus on the positive things that you can do, such as choosing appropriate food items and exercising.

Chapter 6: Protein Absorption During Metabolic Autophagy

Protein is an important part of any diet that you have or will be attempting for yourself, and it plays an important part in autophagy and how it affects your body and cells. In this chapter, we will be looking at how the protein gets absorbed in metabolic autophagy. There are many different studies that have been done on protein and the effects that it has on the human body. There are also just as many studies that attempted to learn how our protein intake has an effect on autophagy and how autophagy might benefit you or become more useful due to how it reacts or interacts with the protein. Most studies were done on protein, you may think, have only been done at the fitness level, but many more are being conducted in new fields now.

As there have been many studies done about how protein works, experts also debate whether or not it is safe for the body. Protein is such a big part of fasting, which is one of the things that is said to be able to activate autophagy. You'll need to understand how it is that your body will be responding to this and how it will be able to work with protein.

We know that the molecules in our body are destined to be discarded, and they are marked with a small protein called ubiquitin. This is recognized by a receptor that's located at the gateway to the proteasome. In this way, it is natural to suggest that there is a similar recognition mechanism for protein degradation by the autophagosomes, according to research and studies that have been conducted over the last thirty years.

Studies that have been conducted internationally on mice have found that they've been able to identify a new protein, in addition to the protein that we already know of. This new protein may act as a receptor, and there are also proteins that are being discovered that are associated with cancer. However, the proteins that are being studied have chain-like structures, which means at one end, they bind to the ubiquitin that marks the protein aggregates and organelles that are to be degraded. Next to this site, where the binding is taking place, is a domain that will bind to other proteins that are found in the autophagosomes membrane. It is here the protein waste can dock on to autophagosomes and can then be wrapped up in the membrane.

The levels of protein within cells are determined not only by the rates of synthesis but also by rates of degradation. The half-lives of proteins within cells are widely varied and can last from minutes to several days. There are also differential rates of protein degradation, and they are an important aspect of cell regulation. Degraded proteins are rapidly degraded function as a regulatory molecule, such as transcription factors. This means that the rapid turnover of these proteins is necessary to allow their levels to change quickly in response to external stimuli.

Because protein is very important to your body and your health, we have compiled some data to make you more aware of just how it affects your body. For example, an error or a kind of failure in the function of a protein can lead to serious diseases, such as prion diseases, where your brain is going to degenerate to a structure that looks like a sponge. This can also cause Alzheimer's, not to mention, cancer. Another fact for you to be aware of is that the human body possesses more than 100,000 proteins of various kinds, and the body utilizes them for different purposes, such as healing and growth. More importantly, they carry out almost all chemical reactions that take place in the body, also for different purposes.

When the proteins possess all nine amino acids that the body is able to produce, they are deemed "complete proteins." These proteins come from a variety of sources, such as meat (poultry, fish, and cattle). "Incomplete proteins" are usually found in nuts and vegetables. If you have a protein deficiency, this can lead to a serious health problem for you, so it's a good idea to make sure that you are getting the proper amount. A good example of a protein deficiency is the Kwashiorkor condition that is common among children. This condition is characterized by the discoloration of the skin, physical effects on the hair (thinning and discoloration), and weight loss. If you leave it untreated, a child with this condition may not grow as he or she should. In extreme cases, it might lead to death.

Facts like these remind us that protein, obviously, plays a very big part in our body, and understanding this is going to help us how to better absorb it and how it can create and trigger autophagy. This is another example of how important protein is for your body. A single protein named albumin can cause the entire human body to swell if you don't have it in your body. It is hard to determine the lifespan of proteins; however, recent studies have been able to show that for most proteins, lifespan is around two days if not shorter, although studies also show that there are some proteins that may live for an extremely long time. Studying these, in particular, experts find that they could have something to do with cell aging and neurodegeneration.

To understand how important protein is, you should think about it like this. Your body is mostly made of water; however, as protein is so involved in the cells of your body, your body is believed to have about twenty percent of protein by weight.

Protein deficiency is rare if you're living in a developed country, even if you are on a vegetarian diet. If you are on a vegetarian diet, you will typically be provided with all the protein that your body needs, even if the diet only includes plant food (which, as a vegetarian, you should be eating anyway, in the absence of meat). As long as you have a wide variety of these foods, you should be alright. However, even though protein is important for your body, and we've talked about the dangers of not having enough, it can also be dangerous to have too much in your system. This may be surprising as we've already been establishing that our bodies need protein and that our bodies are actually made up of a lot of protein, which is all true. However, if you have a high level of protein in your body and it is too much, they can actually stress your liver and your kidneys because they both have to work harder to break down and get rid of the excess protein that you have ingested and absorbed. Another problem with extra protein is that it can cause you to put on weight, which causes an entirely new set of issues for your body.

The proteins in our bodies have many different jobs. A good example would be a protein called rhodopsin. This protein is in our eyes, and its job is to help us to see the light. Another example would be hemoglobin, which is a component of red cells that are distributed from the lungs, carrying the much-needed oxygen for the cells of the body. Aside from that, as it travels through the bloodstream, it collects wastes for discarding.

The protein, in a chain of chemical processes can actually make your blood clot, which can be extremely dangerous. Additionally, other jobs that proteins provide for our body are the following.

- They give the body structure.
- They defend against diseases.
- They help us maintain our body's internal environment.
- They may help to give us energy.
- They help regulate our body's processes that take place on a daily basis.

Insufficient protein or intake of those amino acids can also have an effect on the rest of your body, and this includes the following things:

- Your bone cell synthesis
- Your heart cell turnover rate
- Your red blood cell production
- And many more issues that could seriously plague your body, including organ function

If you're an elderly person, you are also more prone to experiencing body break down extensively, compared to younger people. This makes it a necessity to have more protein in your body; however, as a person transitions to middle-age years, a certain component, the hydrochloric acid, falls to approximately 50 percent. This acid assists in the digestion of proteins in the stomach, so with less of this, older people get less proteins. Cell regeneration is a process that needs proteins in order to take place. With lesser proteins, the cells will have a hard time regenerating. Some experts have been suggesting that aging could be a phenomenon caused by the decrease of protein alone

As a macronutrient, protein is one of the components of our body that provides energy. To be specific, it provides about four calories per gram. Our carbohydrates deliver the same amount, while fats supply about nine calories. Researchers have also been studying alterations in protein that may increase a person's risk of autism. This is a very sensitive subject, and it has been a debate for years. As such, researchers in recent years have begun to believe that a protein called the shank 3 mutates, and when it does, it could lead to defects in neuron communication.

Researchers have also studied Americans, and they believe that they intake almost double the amount of protein that might actually require for growth and other necessities. Also, they believe that middle-aged women or older meet the minimum required amount only, while children are usually below the ideal range. This is one of the reasons that protein needs to be monitored.

One of the great ways that protein can work in fasting and intermittent fasting, which is another topic that we've been studying in this book, is that protein can help make you feel more satiated. This means it is helping you maintain a healthy weight, but protein can also help you feel full. The ability to feel full is something that is going to help you with fasting, as it will help with hunger pains. Just make sure that you're staying within the right amount, and you're not getting too little. Also, make sure that you are not getting too much. Protein is something that really needs to be monitored, which is why having a medical professional is going to help you understand where you need to be.

It is also worth noting that proteins from animal food sources (e.g., chicken, fish, and cow, among others) are more like our proteins compared to the plant proteins. Because of this, the proteins from animal sources are used more rapidly and readily. Studies have shown that it might be easier for our bodies to absorb animal proteins than plant proteins, although both can be absorbed. More studies are being conducted on this because it's a very hot debate, and it's an issue that tends to go back and forth. But studies have shown that the human body readily uses animal protein, actually marginally better than the proteins from plant sources (e.g., nuts). A downside to this, however, is that a lot of types of meat are laden with fat, especially the saturated, unhealthy kind of fat. Therefore, a better type of meat (if you're trying to get your protein from meat) is low in saturated fat and lean. For this, you would have to search for such protein sources.

One downside to some protein sources is the reality of allergies. Certain types of proteins can cause an allergic reaction to certain people—not everyone. (Some people are actually lucky not to have any allergy.) These allergies are a result of the protein's unique structure that could prompt an immune response. An example of this to help make it easier to see and understand is to think of someone who has a food allergy in the form of gluten. If you are allergic to gluten, get protein from other grains and wheat.

The other major pathway of protein degradation involves the uptake of proteins by what is known as a lysosome. A lysosome is a membrane-enclosed organelle that contains an array of digestive enzymes that includes what is called proteases. The containment of proteases prevents uncontrolled degradation of the cell's contents. Therefore, in order to be degraded by this process, the cellular proteins must first be taken up by the lysosomes. One pathway for this uptake of cellular proteins is autophagy, which involves the formation of the autophagosomes, where there are small areas of cytoplasmic organelles that are being enclosed in membranes.

You may not know this, but many of your hormones and enzymes are predominantly protein in nature, which makes it a vital substance in our body. It's also important for repairing and maintaining tissues in the body. However, not all types of protein are equal, and there are ways for you to aid your body to absorb it more efficiently for the different roles that they have in the body. Protein, as we have mentioned earlier in this chapter, is a macronutrient. It is composed of smaller components called amino acids. The body needs twenty of them, but only nine can be produced.

There are other amino acids that you need that you can only get through your diet. This is why whole foods like fish and eggs are recommended for people who need protein. They are good sources for you to ingest, and they will be good for your body and health. Nuts, beans, and seeds are recommended for getting your protein, particularly if you are a vegetarian. The amount of protein that you need is different from person to person because each person has different health needs, and each person is on a different health regimen. It is difficult to understand how much protein a single person needs in a day, but there are ways that you can learn how much protein you need in every day, and your doctor or your nutritionist would be a good person to ask how much protein you should be eating.

Protein digestion begins when you first start eating. Once a protein source reaches your stomach, the acid in your stomach and the enzymes break it down into smaller chains of amino acids. Then the amino acids are joined together with peptides, and they are broken into what is called protease. When this is in your stomach, the smaller chains move into your small intestine. When this happens, your pancreas release enzymes and a buffer that will reduce the acidity of the food that you've digested.

The reduction allows even more enzymes to work on further breaking down the amino acid chains into individual amino acids. Then it's ready to be absorbed, which is what this chapter is about. Protein absorption happens in your small intestine as well because the small intestine contains microvilli. Microvilli are very small structures that are finger-like and that are able to increase the absorbing surface area of your small intestine. So what this does for you is it allows for maximum absorption of the amino acids and other nutrients that you're digesting. Once they have been absorbed, the amino acids are released into your bloodstream, and once they're released into your bloodstream, they are taken to cells in other areas. They do this so that they can start building muscle or repairing tissue.

Through an older study performed, it was thought that proteins from vegetarian sources could be consumed during a single meal in order for the body to form the proteins to complete. This theory has changed since then, and it's been shown that the body is able to pool proteins from a variety of foods throughout the day to form the complete proteins that you need to absorb.

There are also things that you can do for yourself to make your protein absorb better for your body, and they include the following.

- Make sure you chew thoroughly.
- Eat the protein staggered throughout the day instead of all at once.
- Exercise regularly (this helps autophagy too).
- Reduce your stress.
- Avoid intensive exercise right after a meal.

Because protein is a vital nutrient for your whole body, it is digested by your mouth, your stomach, and your small intestine before it is released to your bloodstream. You can maximize your protein intake with the tips above, and by doing so, you can ensure that protein is absorbed properly to trigger autophagy properly as well.

Chapter 7: How to Do Fasting

Fasting is a big trend right now, and the best thing that you can do for yourself is to understand how to do this safely and have the proper information. One of the first things that you need to remember is to stay hydrated, which means you need to drink enough water to stay healthy. While you fast, you may experience some serious side effects like dehydration. Fasting can also result in dry mouth, fatigue, headache, and thirst, so it's very important that you're drinking enough fluids to maintain your health especially since you're fasting and not ingesting anything else.

Most health authorities recommend that you drink eight 8-ounce glasses per day. However, if you are concerned that you're not drinking enough, there are many mobile phone apps that will make sure you're staying hydrated, and many of them tell you exactly how much you should be drinking based on your weight and other important factors. Many of them can actually be fun and innovative, so it seems like you're not just drinking water as a chore but as a game, which makes it easy to do and fun, while helping you remember easily.

However, the actual amount of fluid that you need can vary from person to person because each person is different, and they have their own issues or problems. You get around twenty to thirty percent of the fluid that your body needs from the food that you eat. In a fast, however, you're not eating. As such, it's quite easy to get dehydrated. During a fast, many people actually might need anywhere from eight to fourteen cups of water over the course of a single day because you're depleting your body of what it needs. This is one of the biggest reasons that fasting is unhealthy. To avoid dehydration, your thirst will tell you when you need to drink more. You need to listen to your body and what it is trying to tell you about its needs.

Going for walks can help because it can take your mind from what you're doing. One way of avoiding breaking your fast is to make sure that you're keeping busy with activities that distract from your hunger but don't take up too much energy. An activity should not be too strenuous but is effective enough to keep your mind engaged. You could also take a bath, read a book, or watch a favorite movie—anything that keeps your mind off it.

Another thing that you need to remember is that you need to keep your fasting short. There are many different ways to fast, as there fitness trends popping up left and right, and everybody comes up with a different method of doing so. However, most are unsafe, and therefore, popular methods of fasting need to be evaluated carefully so that you can be safe. Each of them has its own rules, and most are regimented by short fasts that range between eight to twenty-four hours. Some people choose to undertake much longer fasts that range from a day to three days, which is obviously a much longer fast. Doing a fast for this long increases your risk for the following issues.

- Irritability
- Fainting
- Hunger
- Dehydration

There are, unfortunately, even more serious health problems, depending on the medical conditions that you have or the shape that your body is in.

The best way that you can avoid these side effects is to stick to a shorter fasting period of a single day. This is especially true if you're just starting out and you have never done a fast before. It is a necessity that if you are going to do a fast longer than a day, then you will, of course, need to seek medical attention, and make sure that your doctor is with you and watching you the entire time to make sure that you are safe. This is also true of one-day fasts since the art of fasting has been proven that it's not entirely safe. We will be talking about this so that you can be as informed as possible.

Because they are not proven to be safe, it is imperative to inform your doctor and that they are available to help you. It's an important reminder for many because many people think that they can handle this and not need any help when, in fact, they do need supervision by a medical professional.

In general, since fasting involves the removal of some or all foods for a period of time, an important thing that you need to remember is that you can actually eat a small amount of food on fast days. You can opt not to eat on fast days, but some fasting patterns actually allow you to consume up to a quarter of your calorie regimen in a day with food. In this case, if you want to attempt fasting, you can start out small on the days that you have chosen to fast for yourself. This may be a safer action than doing the full-blown fast. By ingesting food, you're helping your body reduce some of the risks associated with fasting, such as the following.

- Fainting
- The feeling of being unfocused
- The feeling of being hungry

It may also make fasting more sustainable for you because you won't feel as hungry, although a warning that needs to be said is that restricting your calories this much in such a drastic way can lead to eating disorders and other issues that can severely harm your body. That said, take extreme precaution when undergoing this diet regimen.

Our next tip for fasting is to make sure that you're not breaking fasts with a feast. It can be extremely tempting after a period of not eating to celebrate with a huge meal and to stuff yourself beyond your reasonable capacity. Breaking your fast with a feast is not a good idea for the following reasons.

- It can lead you to feel bloated.
- It will lead you to feel tired.
- It will lead you to get sick.

In addition, if you're trying to lose weight, feasting can harm your long-term goals because it's going to slow down or even stop your weight loss, and if you're fasting to lose weight, then you need to understand that fasting is not the best way to do this as it leads to health issues. Because your overall calorie quota impacts your weight, if you are consuming all of these excess calories by having a feast after your fast, it is going to reduce your calorie deficit by a big number. The best thing to do to break a fast is to continue eating normally and then get back into the regular eating routine that you had before starting the fast.

Making sure that you are eating enough protein is important as well. This is something to think about when you're attempting to lose weight. When you fast, you lose muscle. Because of this, you need to make sure that you are eating enough protein on your break.

In addition, if you let yourself eat small amounts of food on the fast days, including protein, it can help you handle the hunger pains. This will also ensure that you're getting the proper amount of protein on the days that you're letting yourself eat. It has been shown in studies (though there is a debate) that if you are able to consume thirty percent of your calories in a day from protein, you can significantly reduce your appetite.

On the days when you're not fasting, you should also eat whole foods. If you choose to fast, you still need to be healthy on the days that you're not doing so. Because of this, you will need to make sure that you are eating whole foods on the days that you eat. If you eat a healthy diet of whole foods, studies have shown that such a diet is linked to many different health benefits.

- Cancer
- Chronic illnesses
- Heart disease

Other diseases can happen to you, as well. Foods that are considered whole foods are the following.

- Legumes
- Fruits
- Vegetables
- Fish
- Meat
- Eggs

You may need to consider supplements. This is something that we will go into later in more detail, but for now, we will say that fasting makes you lose essential nutrients that you need for your body. This is because you're not eating, and eating fewer calories than your body needs causes your body not to meet its nutritional needs. It has been proven in studies that people following weight-loss fads and diets are shown to be deficient in many different nutrients. Those who are attempting to fast may need to keep in mind that you will need to consider taking a multivitamin to prevent deficiencies. The nutrients should be gained from food, however.

Tea has actually been shown to help in intermittent fasting because it reduces hunger pains, especially when you're just starting out on a fast. Tea can help alleviate these hunger pains, and these are kinds of tea with catechins, particularly green tea.

Green tea also helps normalize levels in your body so you can fast with fewer problems. Also, it shows great promise when it comes to lowering bad cholesterol, as well as burning the visceral abdominal fat. The former type of fat is believed to be the most unhealthy fat that can be found in organs, such as intestines and liver. It has been called 'active fat' because it can boost one's health risks, including insulin resistance. This is something that fasting, autophagy, and foods like green tea can help with.

Moreover, there are studies saying that green tea can promote autophagy in your system. This is probably why intermittent fasting and green tea are often linked to the concept of anti-aging. Many people also fast to detoxify their body, but there's no actual proof that it can do so. Tea is a unique substance because of the anti-oxidants contained in the leaves. They are also known to rid your system of free radicals, resulting in better health and glowing skin. They also boost mental clarity, as well as your immune system. A good source of polyphenols, tea is considered a natural prebiotic. Remember that you can only experience these detoxification benefits if you drink green tea regularly.

There are different teas that enhance intermittent fasting, and we will discuss them here as well. We have talked about green tea, which is considered one of the healthiest beverages around the world. It's also the second most-consumed drink after water. This makes sense as our bodies are mostly made of water, and we need water more than any other drink to stay hydrated. Obviously, you should go for water first, and if you're drinking tea, go for green tea. One study has shown that your daily calorie expenditure might increase even a bit by drinking green tea. When taken on a daily basis, that small increment is magnified. In addition, the catechins it contains can alleviate ghrelin levels that can suppress cravings for food, especially sugars. However, there are certain health issues which might restrict your green tea intake—ask your doctor, to be safe. Otherwise, you can have up to four cups a day.

Another type of tea is black tea. Like green tea, it is a potent prebiotic that supports your gut health. It promotes a balanced microbiome in your gut and increases the rate by which you reach the autophagy state because of the caffeine it contains. Speaking of caffeine, it can give you a boost during the difficult parts of your fast. Also, the compounds in black tea, according to studies, promote heart health and detoxification, and it might be able to help reduce your stress levels. It also contains an ingredient which could boost your serotonin levels and promote relaxation and better mood.

Ginger tea is also easy on your stomach and can make the stomach feel better by helping your hunger pains. It also has the added benefits of improving your immunity and digestion. Medical professionals around the globe say that drinking at least three cups each day for your health would be beneficial. Most people prefer their tea cold; others prefer it hot.

Mint tea is great for calming your stomach while also being a nice and tasty treat. A calm stomach will also help you complete your fasting better because you won't be plagued by your stomach having issues and causing your mind to focus on your stomach. The other health benefits of mint tea include the ability to reduce pain as well as eliminating inflammation in your body; inflammation can cause hormonal imbalances that cause other health issues in the future. Another great benefit of mint tea is its calming properties, especially when you're stressed. It can also eliminate bad breath, which is a common effect of fasting.

Hibiscus tea not only looks pretty, but it also tastes great. It can help detoxify your liver. This tea helps with inflammatory problems, digestion, and immune system. One of the best benefits of this tea is its role in lowering blood pressure. This is an issue increasingly on the rise even in younger people, and understanding how to avoid this is the reason for the numerous studies conducted.

If you are pregnant, however, none of these teas should be consumed until you get a go signal from a medical professional.

Again, one reason that people choose to fast is the health benefits. Studies show that those who fast also lower their risk of heart disease, diabetes, and insulin resistance. There are less than a handful of these studies that supported these findings, which isn't exactly the best number to go by. Regardless of this, research can show that fasting for a single day (if you do it once a month) may be able to prevent heart disease or insulin resistance, but, as we have mentioned before, consult your doctor first. Doctors usually recommend a fast of twice a year only, and it depends on your health condition.

When choosing between fasting or continuous calorie restriction, it was fasting that was said to be better at insulin resistance reduction because fasting promotes the breakdown of glucose faster, while it decreases the production of insulin. This process would allow your pancreas to rest. In addition, most experts believe that fasting, particularly intermittent, is beneficial because it trains your system to be efficient when burning fat. One research said that fasting could promote the production of human growth hormone by such a wide margin. These hormones are released by the body in times of starvation in order to prompt the burning of fat stores to use as fuel, thereby conserving your lean muscle mass. As this happens, it means your fat cells are reduced; it means you improve weight loss.

It's very important to remember that your exercise regimen should be kept to a mild amount because if you don't, you will end up hurting yourself, and this is something that can cause damage. It's important to listen to your body, especially when it's struggling.

Also, it's important to note that when you fast, you need to understand that for each day you fast, you need at least two days of food to recover what you have lost. There are no studies published at this time that have proven that fasting is safe to do for an extended period of time, however.

On the other hand, you should focus on the known benefits, such as less insulin resistance and those mentioned before, though studies are yet to be conclusive.

Many people have been trying to find a cure for cancer, and scientists are now looking into periods of fasting to see if it can cure cancer or help make a cure possible. They have studied this on mice, and according to the study, they are attempting to establish the evidence that it can mitigate the cell division rate. Experts agree that nutrient deprivation may be causing the growth factors to decrease. Mice are different from humans, especially with metabolism, but if these studies are progressing, others will soon follow.

Again, most people who believe that fasting is a good regimen want to lose weight. For such an endeavor to be successful, there are two things you can do—eat healthily and exercise regularly. This will give you a sustainable healthy body. Another thing is fasting, which will jumpstart your weight loss, but this is not sustainable. It's not something you can keep doing anyway; the doctors only recommend fasting twice a year, as mentioned earlier.

When you fast, your body's initial response is breakdown the glucose in your body. When the glucose has been used up, your system will turn to your fat stores to keep giving you energy for your day-to-day activities. This process is called the state of ketosis, and this is the reason that people follow the ketogenic diet.

However, medical professionals said that this diet was only invented in the first place to help people who suffer from epilepsy. In these cases, the patients were under constant care and supervision, and they didn't stay on this diet for years. They also said that unless you are in extreme circumstances, this diet should not be attempted in any way. If you have permission from your doctor to start this diet, as some do recommend it, then you can follow the ketogenic diet. Your doctor will probably not recommend you doing it for more than 6 months, so take note of that. Otherwise, you might experience untold damage to your body. Staying in ketosis could also bring on a condition known as ketoacidosis. Ketoacidosis is something that can be fatal, especially for diabetes patients. It has been shown that when a diabetic is in this condition and left untreated, they could possibly lose their life in less than an hour. As such, the ketogenic diet should be avoided by people with diabetes.

Intermittent fasting is also being looked into as a way to encourage a healthy diet or a healthy immune system. Because this is such a hot topic, researchers have been able to show that those who are fasting stick to natural foods, like vegetables and fruits with high-water content, instead of processed ones. For this reason, they believe that fasting would encourage healthy eating choices. If you're into intermittent fasting combined with a healthy, balanced diet, then you can boost your immunity to diseases and infections.

Perhaps one of the biggest reasons that people attempt to fast, besides weight loss, is the belief of detoxifying the digestive system, giving it a rest. Your organs process your food intake, working nonstop, but when you fast, those busy organs get a break since you're not eating anything. On an intermittent fasting schedule, you eat meals on your off days, and then your organs rest again on your fasting window. This is believed to help your digestive system and let it heal.

Because there are so many different side effects that the medications these days have on your body, which could possibly cause more damage than what it's trying to solve, choose natural methods. Undergoing a healthy diet and the intermittent fasting method would be a non-invasive and safe way of fighting against blood pressure and similar health issues, such as the risk of arteries being blocked by fat. This is another reason that people have been looking into fasting and why more research has been conducted on the subject. When you fast, your body signals the use of fat stores to burn as energy since you are not taking any food.

All these factors work together to keep your limits regulated, as well as your metabolic rate. This causes an overall reduction in your blood pressure.

Brain function is another issue that many people are worried about since neurodegenerative diseases are on the rise. Research has shown that intermittent fasting can provide a much-needed boost by increasing the rate of BDNF production. The protein BDNF is known for activating the stem cells in your brain to convert into new neurons. This protein protects your brain cells in the event of a neurodegenerative disease, which can alter them. It will also help prevent your neuromuscular system from degenerating. Fasting would be something to look into to prevent such a disease, as long as it's done safely and healthily.

Another note to mention is that people who were saved from something like famine, for example, is at risk of sudden death if they are suddenly given a lot of food. This is what is called refeeding syndrome. Most people are healthy before fasting, so for them, it would take a couple of weeks for a possible refeeding syndrome to pose a risk. However, if you have fasted or went on a certain diet before, you are on a certain age, or you have an illness, then you should be aware that this will shorten the interval before the risk of sudden death begins. Many people are not aware that refeeding is dangerous, but it is, and it's something that you need to be aware of for your body.

It's also been shown that assertions that our bodies can conserve its functional tissue in an effective manner and our metabolic resting rate across days of fasting (especially total fasting) is based on ideology and not science. In particular, it is not based on solid science. Fasting can also affect your metabolism, as well, and this isn't always a good thing either. Studies show that a healthy diet and exercise are still better to achieve weight loss and good health for your body, and they have both been proven to be safer than fasting. There is also no evidence to support that fasting will detoxify your body. This is a matter of serious debate, but as of yet, there is no scientific evidence to support the claims.

Chapter 8: When You Shouldn't Fast

There are many times that you shouldn't fast, and we will discuss that in-depth here as fasting can be very dangerous for many people. There has been no scientific evidence that fasting is good for you, but people do it for many different reasons. There are medical reasons for fasting; some religions have fasting involved in them, so their followers feel the need to fast for different reasons. Some people fast because of weight loss reasons; however, there is no evidence to support that this will actually help you. In some cases, it can hurt you. This is what we're going to talk about in this chapter.

Fasting is not advisable for everyone, especially those with medical conditions that don't respond to other treatments. It will hurt people that have renal insufficiency or hepatic insufficiency. It will hurt those with a history of cardiac arrhythmias and people with wasting diseases or malnutrition, and it will especially hurt pregnant women and their unborn child.

Anyone who fasts for extended periods should also do so under supervision, as it's not safe. It is not advisable to fast if you have diabetes (in any form) as this can be a dangerous problem and lead you to get hurt. An example of what we meant is that if you have diabetes, and you are trying to regulate it with medicine from your doctor. When you don't eat your carbs, and you stop them for a day, you will be causing your body to change how much medication you need for that day. What could happen then is that the body's response to the medications can be altered, and it will set off your blood glucose in a threatening way. This could cause damage to you internally because of the spikes.

If you have a physically demanding job, you're going to find that you have a big reduction in your performance in all areas. If you already have marginal levels of important minerals in your body, then the problem with people who have diabetes is taking medications. They can get seriously hurt because it causes their bodies to act up when they need to be within a certain regulated regime. For diabetic people, their blood sugar and insulin need to stay within a certain range for them to be healthy, and if it spikes too high or too low, it can cause issues like ketoacidosis, which can be fatal.

Another reason that should prevent you from fasting is pregnancy. If you are pregnant or trying to become pregnant, you cannot go without food for long hours. When you're pregnant, the only thing that you should be focusing on is your unborn child and making sure that you are as healthy as possible. Fasting has been shown to harm the unborn child, as well as the mother. When the baby is in your womb, the baby needs as many nutrients as possible, and you need to maintain a good level of health so that the pregnancy goes safely, and the baby is born healthily without any problems. By starving your body, you are also starving your child of the nutrients that it needs to develop properly.

Another time that you should not fast is if you're immunosuppressed. There is an interesting research study that has focused on the benefits of fasting for people who were undergoing certain issues, but more studies needed to be performed to be accurate. It has been shown, however, that you should never undergo fasting if you're experiencing the following issues.

- Battling cancer
- If you have HIV
- If you have AIDS

- If you have any other immunosuppressive element
- If you are on chemotherapy
- If you're under eighteen years old

In the case of being under the age of eighteen, studies have shown that intermittent fasting is not safe because your bodies are still developing, and your brains are still developing. Also, there are many negative aspects of fasting if you're under eighteen; it can cause issues for your health at an early age.

Children are still developing physically and mentally, and they don't need to have any nutritional stress. Although the occasional fasting has been studied in adults, formative childhood years should not be played with, and it's been shown to be dangerous to ages under eighteen. Humans have higher levels of certain things to help them grow and develop properly, and this is the reason that fasting under the age of eighteen is never advised because you need higher levels of what your body is supplying for you to stay healthy.

You should also never fast if you have an eating disorder. If you have an eating disorder, you are already putting your body through untold damage that can include rotting teeth, esophagus tears, a damaged heart, damaged internal organs, undernourished brain, and many more, depending on the type of eating disorder that you have. Fasting can only harm your body further. Fasting is only going to exacerbate those problems and cause more harm to your body. It could even cause death. As such, it is strongly advised by medical professionals that eating disorder patients do not fast at all, and even when they are in recovery, it is advised that they do not fast as it could put them in negative mind space, and it could trigger them.

Intermittent fasting also has been proven unsafe, as it can cause negative side effects like the following.

- Anxiety
- Stress
- Hair loss

Fasting, in general, can give rise to orthorexia. Orthorexia has been classified as an eating disorder in recent years, and it involves an obsession with healthy eating. A large sign that this is leading to an eating disorder is when your diet becomes inflexible, and if you're already obsessed with healthy eating, fasting is said to be something that you want to avoid as it could lead to a more dangerous situation with your disorder.

Having this issue is going to worsen your disorder. Eating disorders are very unsafe, to begin with, and anything that's going to take it further should be avoided. Fasting can also disrupt your sleep, and this can cause other issues to your health because the quality of your sleep improves things for your body and mind such as the following.

- Your learning capacity
- Your memory
- Your mood
- And other aspects of your health

Also, there are dangerous side effects, such as making you less aware or alert. This is particularly dangerous if you're driving a car or if you're operating machinery. If you're a doctor, for example, you need to be alert. Otherwise, you might not perform well in operation, for instance. Now, this might be seen as an extreme example, but it has been recorded that accidents have been made in professional fields when the professional wasn't alert. The reason that fasting can lead to decreased alertness is that your body is not consuming enough calories, and it's not providing you with adequate energy.

It can also provide people with guilt, which is a negative aspect of this and a reason why people shouldn't do it. When people give themselves a window for eating or fasting, and they feel guilty about breaking it, the resulting issue is that it causes anxiety and shame. Because of these things, it could even cause self-loathing or self-hatred.

These are all things that need to be avoided; no one should hate themselves, and no one should be ashamed of themselves. This can cause lifelong mental disorders and mental issues, along with eating disorders. Fasting can also increase your levels of cortisol, which makes you more stressed. The additional stress can lead to other health issues. If you fast on an unhealthy level, people may also feel colder as a result of lower blood sugar. If you are a woman, fasting can cause you to miss your period. It could also cause irregular periods. Having irregular periods may not seem like it would be that much of an issue now, but in the future, it could cause infertility, and it can cause other issues with your bodies as well. Fasting can also cause (in certain cases) the following.

- Anxiety
- Depression
- Anti-social feelings

If you notice that you are feeling *hangry* (which is a cross between hungry and angry, and it has been proven to be a real issue), this is another time that your body is trying to tell you that maybe you should stop, and you need to pay attention to it.

Humans need fuel to stay healthy, so you need to listen to what your body is saying that it needs and not do a hard fast when your body can't handle it. An issue to worry about is that you are not getting nutrients when you're starving your body and not letting yourself eat. The lack of fuel or energy for your daily activities can make you sick.

Fasting is also not a good idea for people who are highly active, as you will not be giving yourself the fuel that you need. Highly active people attend to consume more calories than people who are not because they are using their bodies a lot for specific activities. As such, they need the fuel and the energy to keep going so they can keep up the regime that they are used to. If you're fasting, then you should be keeping your exercise mild at best, so this wouldn't be a good idea for an active person because there's no way that they would get the fuel that they need to balance out the exercise. For these people, fasting would damage their body or cause them to get hurt from nutrient loss and other damages.

People who take prescription medication are also people who shouldn't fast, as it can cause your medication to react in a negative way. If you're a woman who has a history of amenorrhea, you also should not fast.

Caffeine is an issue with fasting, as well as most intermittent fasting plans. These plans allow you to drink it. As it is one of the few things that you can eat, you could find yourself gravitating toward this stimulant that keeps you going for hours on end. This is dangerous as it ups your levels of cortisol and seriously effects your sleep patterns. Even a tiny increase in cortisol, such as those that you would get from drinking caffeine, can raise your blood sugar, and it will increase the resistance to insulin. Caffeine is also linked to causing depression and anxiety (in many cases).

Fasting also increases inflammation and food intolerances. When you fast, you get into a famished state, and you become more susceptible to the refeeding syndrome. This might lead you to eat unhealthy foods or binge when you break your fast.

All of these issues are occasions when you should not fast. Fasting when you shouldn't has the potential to be fatal; it can cause issues and conditions that could be worse than what you are already facing. This is why many doctors advise against it and explain the proper ways to get healthy without compromising your health or well-being.

Chapter 9: Types of Meals You Should Consume

This chapter will be discussing the meals that you can have on an autophagy diet and, later on in this chapter, an intermittent fasting diet. As mentioned before, this has not been proven safe, so please see your doctor before attempting this in any form.

In autophagy, when you are eating for the first four days a week, you may eat fat and protein for breakfast and end your day with carbs. Snacks are permitted as well. You are allowed one midmorning snack that is high in protein and one carbohydrate-rich snack late in the afternoon. For those who worry about missing out on their sweets, you are allowed a moderate amount of dark chocolate (a single ounce).

The autophagy diet recommends whole foods. In itself, whole foods are not particularly dangerous, as many types of diet endorse them; it's the timing and amount of food that you eat that is said to be potentially harmful to your body. It can result in major health issues and risks (particularly among diabetics).

Having carbs in the morning is going to trigger a flood of insulin. This flood is going to cause your body to hold on to fat. This is amplified when cortisol peaks in the morning. For the autophagy diet, it is important that you eat your carbs at night because your cortisol level is going to be at its lowest and your body is getting ready for bed. It is believed that by boosting your serotonin, your carbs should help induce a soporific and relaxed state. The hard part is said to be the three nonconsecutive days a week where you fast for sixteen hours so that you can kick start your autophagy. A good example is when you eat your nightly meal. For this example, if you eat dinner at seven at night, for instance, you wouldn't be able to eat again until eleven in the morning the next morning.

On your fasting days, you also eat less protein, so you are depriving your body of nutrients that it needs. Restricting calories and protein focus your body to burn fat for nourishment, and if you're able to do this properly, it is believed that your body will selectively start to cannibalize on itself. It is then believed that it will feast on the wrinkle and fat-causing debris that float around in the cells of your body. So now, we're going to explain what type of meals you should be eating on this diet.

Some examples of autophagy meals that you can eat on this diet are the following.

Section one would be breakfast:

- Veggie egg omelet
- Protein whey smoothies
- Bacon with fruit slices
- Grapes with boiled eggs (2)

Section two would be lunch:

- Salad greens with any of the following dressings: lemon, avocado, cheese, or olive oil.
  Veggie stir-fry with beef and a chicken wrap

Section three would be dinner:

- Salmon salad (boiled)
- Fish (grilled)
- Baked potatoes with sirloin that is grilled
- Asparagus with grilled chicken
- Chicken curry with bread or tortilla

Now, let's look at some meals that you can have with intermittent fasting.

A sample of different breakfasts that you can eat includes one of the following.

- A smoothie that is eight ounces and contains kale, apple, and spinach
- A quarter of a cup of oatmeal
- A single egg that is hardboiled
- A single egg tex-mex scramble that has only a pinch of salsa, garlic, tomatoes, and onion
- Vanilla protein shake. It has to be vegan.
- A protein shake that is mint chip
- A breakfast bar, as long as it is paleo
- Egg muffins

Sample lunches that you can eat may include one of the following examples.

- A small potato that has been baked. You may add a single spoon of sour cream
- One-half of avocado on toast with a single spoon of sesame seeds or of peanuts that have been crushed.
- A slaw salad. It should be broccoli.

- Taco salad
- Chicken salad with avocado
- Chickpea salad. It will need to be vegan.
- Pita sandwiches made with tuna salad

Sample dinners that you can eat may include one of the following examples. You will notice in the dinner's list that salad and chicken are popular options for you to choose from.

- Two cups of vegetables that have been roasted
- Soup with beans, vegetables, and chicken. It should have a quarter cup of beans with half a cup of vegetables that have been chopped. The chicken should be three ounces. If you don't like chicken, you can substitute it for a small portion of tofu or a piece of buffalo or beef that is three ounces.
- Vegetables with peanut chicken
- Thai chicken salad. Make it a citrus salad.
- Mediterranean quinoa salad
- Mexican quinoa salad. Use tempeh.
- Spicy chicken chili

Sample snacks that you can eat have a variety of things to choose from. These are popular options, and some that may surprise you. Examples include one of the following.

- A quarter to half a banana
- Two cups of microwave popcorn that has been cooked
- Two dozen almonds
- Half a cup of cottage cheese
- A single baked apple
- A quarter cup of ice cream that is low in sugar
- Whole grain pretzel sticks but only three pieces
- One fruit of choice
- Nuts
- Yogurt
- Trail mix
- Edamame
- Zucchini chips

Watching portion sizes is important because this type of diet is all about when you eat; the timing is important and needs to be monitored carefully. As this diet is about not eating more than you are eating, you will notice the portions are a bit small. But once you begin to do this, you will get the hang of it, and it will become easier as you understand the mechanisms.

Other things that you can eat and drink are the following.

- Water. This one is probably obvious, but the reason that we are mentioning it, along with your meals, is that the health of every organ in your body depends on water. When you are fasting, it can be difficult for some people to remember that they need to drink water because they are not eating. You need to remember to drink enough to stay hydrated, and your urine should be a pale yellow or clear and have little to no odor. This is (one of the signs) how you know that you are healthy. You should also stay hydrated. Dark urine (that is yellow; if you have brownish, then that's the sign of a more serious problem like a urinary infection) can cause lightheadedness, headaches, and fatigue. When you are only eating limited food, this could cause you serious health issues. For people who don't like plain water, you can add some lemon juice to your water, which has shown to help with digestion, some cucumber, or mint leaves if that suits you better.

- Eggs are another thing that we have listed above because they are a good source of protein, and they keep you full. Another benefit that they have is the ability to help build muscle. There were studies done showing that men who ate breakfast with eggs instead of something like bagel felt full longer and ate less as the day progressed. This is why if you hard-boil an egg, it's not time-consuming and you are getting a good protein that you need during your fasting.
- We've also talked about veggies, but cruciferous veggies are going to help you better. Cruciferous vegetables are full of fibers. When you're eating sporadically or erratically, you need fiber-rich foods. This is vital to make sure that you are not constipated when you are fasting. Another thing that fiber will do for you is to make sure that you are feeling full, and this is something that you will need if you are going to refrain from eating for sixteen hours.

- Avocados are alright here, too. It may seem like it's counterproductive to eat food so high in calories, but the reason that this is alright is that it offers monosaturated fat. It's very satiating, which means that you stay fuller longer, which is something that will help you stay focused on the fast and not break it.
- Probiotics are another thing that you can have while you are performing an intermittent fast. To counteract the issues that arise from fasting (such as stomach issues and constipation), add some foods that are rich in probiotics to your diet.
- If you drink smoothies, then you already know about the health benefits of having fruit in your diet. They are great sources of vitamins and antioxidants, and studies have shown that people who consumed a diet that was rich in flavonoids, such as in strawberries and blueberries, had smaller increases in their body mass index over a period of fourteen years than those who didn't.
- Potatoes are known for being a satiating food. Another study that was performed showed that eating potatoes as a part of your healthy diet can help you lose weight.

- Beans and legumes for chili can be a yummy thing to eat, and the carbs will give you energy. In addition to these foods, peas, black beans, and chickpeas are foods that have been shown to decrease your body weight, even when you are not fasting.
- Nuts are foods that you can also eat. Just be sure you don't go overboard. They are full of good fat, and studies show that it might be possible that the poly fat in walnuts may alter the markers (at least the physiological ones) for satiety and hunger.
- Fish is another good food for you to consume because it's called brain food. As you are restricting your calories and it may alter your cognition, this is a good food to help with that. It is rich in protein and healthy fats, along with ample amounts of vitamin D. This is a great food to eat, especially if you are limiting your food because you're getting a good bang for your buck as far as nutrition goes. It can also help you with your fast to make sure that you are alright.
- Whole grains are rich in protein and fiber; this is why eating a little is going to help you feel full for

a longer period . It can help you in other areas as well. A new study, for example, suggests that if you are eating whole grains instead of the refined grains, it may possibly rev up your metabolism. On a day when you have to restrict so much food because you want to fast for more than half a day, this is going to help you remain fuller so that you can take your mind away from the fact that you are not letting yourself eat the way you normally do.

Other foods that are supposed to stimulate autophagy are the following.

- Coffee
- Green tea
- Elderberries

By using these foods to your advantage, you can have a successful fast.

Chapter 10: Metabolic Autophagy in Terms of Biology and Science

Autophagy is also linked to biology and science, which shouldn't surprise you because at its core, it is considered to be studied by scientists in many different areas. Autophagy serves as a housekeeping function, which we've already talked about in other chapters, and it will help the energy demands balance during the times of stress. The term was shown to us in the last century by a man who was both a biochemist and cytologist. There are three different forms of autophagy, which we've also discussed, and your cells rely primarily on the first one. The way that this relates to biology is the fact that there are many different genes that encode the plethora of components of the autophagy machinery that is needed for many different areas, such as degradation, sequestration, and recycling of your cellular materials. The enzymes are also encoded with a multitude of different genes, and they join together, which enhances your enzyme activity. This is particularly true under the formation of the autophagosome.

There are a number of nonspecific cellular pathways that are also critical to autophagy, and this includes various pathways, such as the endocytic and secretory pathways. In addition to this, the cytoskeleton appears to serve multiple functions in autophagy. One of the key roles among them is the role of microtubules and facilitating autophagosome transport in your mammalian cells.

In addition to the stress response abilities that autophagy is able to perform, autophagy can also contribute to immunity. This is what helps defend your cells against organisms that cause diseases. They then participate in what's known as antigen presentation. Autophagy is also involved in other areas, including programmed cell death, helping eliminate apoptotic cells during what is known as embryonic development or even aiding in the death processes in your cells that are apoptosis defective.

It can also protect you against cell death because it provides your cells with nutrients during periods of starvation. In cancer, autophagy is present as well. It seems to do two things. It seems to prevent tumor progression, and in certain conditions, it promotes tumor progression.

Abnormal accumulation of autophagic vesicles has been associated with many different neurodegenerative conditions. These include conditions like amyotrophic lateral sclerosis, as well as with a disease of skeletal muscle tissue known as myopathy.

Autophagy influences your cells survival through cell bioenergetics and the clearance of the aggregates of protein and organelles that are damaged. There are studies and evidence that have indicated that autophagy is a multifaceted regulator of cell death. Controversy exists on the subject of autophagy in many different ways, such as whether or not autophagy by itself can drive cell death under physiological circumstances that are reverent.

Although autophagy is most evident in the following starvation, there is a basal level of constitutive autophagy that occurs or appears to be a universal feature of certain cells. Autophagy is seemingly at odds with its role in being able to promote cell survival because it's often observed at high levels in dying cells, and in some cases, it can actively contribute to cell death. This can also be referred to as type 2 programmed cell death, and it's different from type 1, which is apoptin cell death.

Although autophagy and cell death are unclear in many cases, it may involve the targeted destruction of factors that you need for cell survival. They also play a part in cell growth and adaptation to stress and starvation.

In general sense, autophagy is a process that is supposed to help your cells. As such, most people use this word synonymously with macroautophagy. In double membrane, bound vesicles will form in the cytosol. From there, it sequesters cytoplasm and fuses with the lysosome. This will release an inner vesicle and the autophagic body into the lumen.

After this happens, the cargoes are then broken down by resident hydrolases. The resulting macromolecules are recycled. Autophagy is generally considered to be non-specific, but there are examples of very specific autophagy that includes the degradation of excess peroxisomes.

Autophagy is unique as a mechanism that can have the ability to remove organelles in their entirety, which is an important task that goes beyond the abilities of the proteasome in the aspect of allowing removal of obsolete organelles or damaged organelles. This potentially eliminates oxidative stress or allows cellular remodeling.

There have been many tests conducted on animals that have had various different results in the facets of biology and autophagy and how they are related. One thing to remember is that although there have been studies that show the merits of autophagy and how it benefits us, it has been proven that more tests and research need to be done for us to have more conclusive knowledge.

There is still plenty that we don't know, and one of the things that we don't know is the source of the membrane that is being sequestered. Many protein components have been identified, but we don't really know the functions of most of them. These limitations are causing issues because we do not know how the vesicle is formed, and this is a big part of macroautophagy (which is one of the most well-known forms of autophagy). Another issue is how specificity is achieved, either for the recognition of invading pathogens or for the removal of a particular organelle.

There is science behind autophagy, as well. The term comes from a Greek term that means self-devouring. As early as three years ago, a Japanese scientist won the Nobel Prize for his discoveries about the mechanisms of autophagy. This has caused drug companies and people in the academic field to want to find something that we can use to stimulate the process, believing that the process can be induced naturally by high-intensity exercise and restricting your carbohydrate intake.

The problem with this is that the only evidence that shows any success is experimenting with mice. As such, it has been proven that this is not enough to go on, and more studies need to be done so that we have better information to use.

In the mid part of the last century, there was a study that was performed through an electron microscope on mouse kidneys. They were newborn, and he spotted something that he had never seen before the test. He saw a membrane-bound structure that was within the cytoplasm of the cells in the kidney. It was interesting that the structures that he saw seemed to contain altered mitochondria.

The man quickly published what he found, and then more independent researchers began to support the findings as well. This was conducted about twelve years after, and they found information regarding cytoplasm. It is known today as macro-autophagy.

One of the things that they discovered is that the formation of a double-membrane structure is transient. This structure was later termed a phagophore. In contrast to the secretory transport vesicles, this one acquires cargo during its assembly.

It may also form what is known as de novo in the cytoplasm as a free-standing structure. It may also be in contact with an organelle. An example of this would be an endoplasmic reticulum. There was more research conducted, and they found that it was the autophagosome that they discovered in the last century.

There are also different categories of autophagy. We have discussed that there are three different kinds of autophagy, but we haven't discussed that there are two other ways that they can be categorized: selective or non-selective. This is based on the nature of what you are eating.

Today, autophagy is recognized as a process for maintaining cellular homeostasis that is vital. It's also for responding to stressors in your body. An example of this would be a nutrient deficiency. This may potentially cause your cell survival to be compromised. When your cells are exposed to stressors like these, autophagy is strongly upregulated. This causes sequestration to increase and the degradation of parts of the cell to release macromolecules back into the cytosol. This is going to power essential metabolic reactions and generate energy.

Autophagy's contribution to the health of your cells under stress conditions and normal conditions implies physiological and pathological roles that are important for this process, which is precisely orchestrated and regulated. Recent research has discovered that autophagy is a critical modulator for a different range of disorders and diseases. Because of this, more research is being done to understand the development of the roles that the pathway's play a part in. As we only partly understand the morphology, along with other key aspects, there is much information that is still emerging and that we can learn from.

The reason that autophagy is unique is that it is flexible in the autophagosome cargo selection and size. Autophagy is compactly regulated, and this is to make sure that it is ramped when it is required to do so. From there, it will be in a manner that is timely. The metabolic sensor of the cell is also known as TOR complex 1, and it is sensitive to the availability of growth factors and amino acids. It also inhibits autophagy induction when the components are plentiful.

When the cells are being deprived of those molecules, your TORC1 inactivates, which promotes an increase in autophagy. Other nutrients can trigger autophagy, as well, particularly when certain nutrients reach critically low levels.

It also plays a key role in development by being instrumental during the course of mammalian development. However, there are problems with autophagy, as well. With the role of autophagy in physiology, dysregulation of the process is tied to many different pathologies, including certain diseases and cancer. Understanding the relationship between them could be important for being able to design therapeutic interventions that are effective.

Studies have been going on for years about autophagy and its benefits to you. They have even performed studies in veterinary medicine for mammalian cells to see how autophagy affects them. Researches have only begun recently to understand how certain cells react to others and how they destroy invading pathogens. Autophagy can work with components of the innate immune system in certain situations, but many studies are still being done to see up to what extent it can perform. More recent work from laboratories and medical colleges have revealed that autophagy in certain forms and in relation to reticulum could be an essential component of a cellular stress response. However, in moderating your immune system, biology may not always be advantageous, as studies have shown that autophagy may play a role in aggravating auto-degenerative diseases like multiple sclerosis and autoimmune diseases that affect the essential nervous system. Autophagy is seen as protective, which is shown by its function in many neurodegenerative disorders, but studies go back and forth repeatedly on how effective it actually is for the human body. Doctors are still performing more research to give more accurate information, and this is especially true since autophagy has been linked to cancer. As a scientific field, the studies about this particular subject encounter a new juncture, and people who are studying autophagy have been able to see some mechanisms related to this, but they haven't uncovered enough. There's still many more questions and even more concerns as well as worries about the functions that this subject performs. There are many more studies being done in physiology and how it relates to autophagy. We know that we have to eat to live, but it's still unclear as to how much autophagy can benefit or hurt us.

In any aspect of a scientific field, we know that the more research we do, the more information that we will find, which is why studies and funding are going into this subject. When we can learn more, we can truly see how autophagy benefits us.

Chapter 11: Metabolic Autophagy While Sleeping

Autophagy is also good for your sleep, or so they say in certain studies. Healthy sleep requires smart thinking, and this is true for all people. No matter what type of sleeper you happen to be, there's a way to get in touch with your circadian rhythm and optimize your autophagy. It's habitual to get into bed and have all your technology with you, but for optimal sleep, you will need to have no technology anywhere near you at least an hour and a half before you go to bed. If you can't live without your phone for helping you sleep, there is software that can reduce the hues from your screen. Orange-tinted glasses or light bulbs will also do the trick. According to sleep doctors, if you set the alarm for an hour before you go to bed, it will give you a reminder that you need to power down. If you power down, you can follow the following rhythms. At the first 15 minutes, you should take care of all the things you have to do before bed and then the things that you usually wait on can be done as well.

In the second quarter, you need to take time for your hygiene needs. A hot shower or a bubble bath will help you sleep because it changes the core body temperature. When you get out of the tub or the shower, it is going to help your body because it starts to relax. The last part of the hour should be taken for relaxation to help you sleep. It is said that the ideal temperature is about sixty-five degrees, and the cooler your body is, the better you're going to sleep. The decrease in your body core temperature is also going to align your body with your circadian rhythm, so the effect is better and more comfortable sleep.

Silence will help you sleep, but many of us live in very large cities or towns that have constant noise. Examples include living near trains and an airport, or you have family members who are still up very late, making sorts of noises when you're about to sleep. Another thing that interferes with sleep is children. This one is obviously something that many people have to deal with during the night, so it's not hard to understand how you would lose sleep here and how it would be harder to get yourself the allotted time to sleep for the sake of your health. Noise produces a sonic noise, and you can determine them by two things: frequency and power or amplitude. You've probably heard of white noise, which includes all the frequencies and supposed colors that come with noise but the combination sounds like static in some cases and other noises in others.

Other noises balance the frequencies a little bit more, and they sound more like falling rain. Different colors have different frequencies, including high frequencies. These frequencies will produce sounds that sound like waves. The noises can help you sleep, and many people find that crashing waves helps them go to sleep faster than other noises. A note, however, is that crashing waves can make others feel that they have to go to the bathroom. While this isn't true for everyone, if you are one of these people, avoiding the waves would be a good idea. But another option is buying a noise machine. Noise machines have many different sounds and mechanisms, so there would be something on them for everyone, and you would find what suits you best and helps you sleep better. If you don't want to spend that kind of money (they range from cheap to very expensive, so it can be a pain trying to find one), there are many apps that you can download for free on your smartphone and help you determine which noises help you fall asleep the best.

But autophagy can help with your sleep through your circadian rhythm. It not only helps control the cycle of your sleep and awake times, but it is also linked to autophagy, as some studies show. Our biological clock can affect the rhythm of autophagy, and getting a proper amount of sleep can actually help you with this. In a study conducted on sleep interruption on mice, they noticed that if the mice were interrupted when they were trying to sleep, it also negatively affected the autophagy.

This is often referred to as sleep disruption. If the protein transmission is interrupted, this causes issues as well. As this was not to be tested on humans, we have no idea what would happen if it affects a human being. More studies need to be conducted, however. But the studies on sleep using mice have shown that sleep and autophagy may be linked.

All living organisms, like humans, for example, have a built-in sleep and wakefulness cycle and circadian rhythm. Believe it or not; they actually coincide with periods of scarcity, meaning feast or famine or food abundance. Autophagy is the process of self-eating, as we discussed earlier, and because of this, the cells in your body begin to disassemble and break all of their dysfunctional components.

Deficient autophagy promotes aging and disease. All of your aged cells will age because of accumulated inflammation, and they will age because of insufficient repair. This is why it's important to understand how autophagy affects your sleep. Circadian rhythms are considered to be your body's psychological process that's connected to the day and night cycles of your environment. This controls metabolism, as well as hormones, brain activity, and epigenetics. If your circadian rhythm is misaligned, it can be linked to metabolic syndrome, depression, obesity, cancer, or even neurodegeneration. This is primarily caused by the blue light exposure in the evening that will disrupt the body's circadian clocks, which interferes with the sleep quality that can get.

Lack of sleep and bad sleep quality can lead to many different health issues, including an increased risk of dying. Getting quality sleep is vital for staying healthy. While asleep, your body goes through many different processes, such as repairing your body, learning new skills, and undergoing autophagy. When your brain clears out what is known as beta-amyloid, along with proteins that are toxic, this can be associated with Alzheimer's.

Autophagy can be modulated with the sleep hormone known as melatonin. Dysfunctional autophagy is also associated with chronic and acute patho-physio behavior, along with neurodegenerative behavior changes. It is approximated than more than half of the pulses of growth hormone occur during deep sleep or what is known as slow-wave sleep. The growth hormones act on the liver, which is meant to stimulate autophagy.

As said before, there haven't been any studies on humans. If you are exercising and utilizing tips to help with your autophagy, but your sleep isn't good, this doesn't mean that you are hopeless. Fasting while you're suffering from sleeping issues is generally considered to be a bad idea, although this is a very hot topic for debate. If you're sleep-deprived, then you are more likely to suffer from metabolic issues, and it is said that fasting affects you metabolically. You should take your quality of sleep seriously, and it is an important step to autophagy. You will be much a healthier person if you fix your sleep around what's important and what you need to do for yourself to improve your health and issues. Correcting your circadian rhythm will improve your cycles, your deep sleep and your body.

When you're trying to get your autophagy to happen or activate when you're sleeping, there are some interesting things that can come into play. The more you know, the better you can understand autophagy. In addition to this, the information can be quite interesting.

Humans are the only mammals that will delay their sleep on purpose, and this isn't healthy because of the fact that you need healthy sleep each night. You should avoid insomnia because if you're not getting healthy sleep, it's going to affect your health in negative ways.

If you live at a high altitude, this affects your sleep in a negative way. The higher the altitude you live at, the greater the chance that you will have sleep disruption. There are ways to make this better because even though you're in a place that affects your sleep, you can still power down and exercise to help your sleep get better and healthier.

Exercising usually makes it easier for people to fall asleep in that it also contributes to sounder sleep. Remember it is said that autophagy, while you're sleeping, is easier to experience and to conduct. When you exercise on a daily basis, it is said to be more helpful to your body because you are making healthier choices. It also helps you become tired naturally.

Caffeine has also been known to affect sleep, and because you're going to be using caffeine to keep you energized and awake while you're fasting or to keep you from feeling hunger pains while you're fasting, this is something to keep in mind. In general, it is said that many adults who are of a healthy nature will need at least seven hours of sleep at night. However, others may need eight, nine, or even more than this. As everyone is different and has different health issues and needs, it is interesting to note that some can perform with less hours of sleep, while others couldn't perform certain activities unless they slept more (around even ten hours which would make others feel groggy and unhealthy).

Another issue to be aware of is that people usually feel tired at various times of the day. But, there are two times of the day, in particular, that affect most people, and they are early in the morning (around two in the morning) and in the midafternoon (around two in the afternoon).

It is natural that we would feel a drip in our alertness during the afternoon, and this is referred to as a post-lunch dip. This is the afternoon crash that most people talk about when you think about people who work in an office area or something like that. Everyone can experience it, though. Students experience it during their last classes of the day and end up crashing when they get home. By taking naps, they tend to have insomnia late at night because they had already napped when they got home.

According to recent studies, there are other issues that can cause sleep issues, which surprisingly include your marital status. If you are divorced, widowed, or separated, it is said that you might be more prone to insomnia than those who are married or in a relationship. If you have these issues, it means that your autophagy might also be messed up. There has been a study performed about the use of melatonin in helping the time it takes to fall asleep, but it's not verified as of yet in many aspects, and other negative issues have been shown.

One thing to be aware of, however, is that melatonin has a habit of reacting to other medications. If you're on medication, you shouldn't take it because it can cause reactions, which can cause underlying problems for you. If you're pregnant or are breastfeeding, you shouldn't take it either because it can be dangerous for both you and your child. It's primarily a good idea to ask your doctor if this would be alright for you to take, and if it is, you might find that you get some help with falling asleep and having a healthy and fuller sleep.

In the United States, it has been shown that one of the biggest reasons that people experience sleepiness is because of the fact that they are depriving themselves of it. Whether it is because of work or children, it seems that Americans stay up much more than they need to and force themselves not to sleep.

This happens in other countries across the globe as well, and it spans across many careers. A good example here is a writer. Writers often get stereotyped as staying up for hours on end and drinking coffee all night. While the coffee isn't true (because who could possibly drink that much coffee), it is proven that they stay awake for hours on end, trying to find another idea or inspiration.

Another example is a doctor. They are always on call, and while they do get sleep, they have to be ready at a moment's notice. The same is true for firefighters, police officers, or military soldiers. Whatever it is, there are millions of people who are forgoing sleep when they need it the most.

In addition to this, because they are not letting themselves fall asleep, they are not triggering autophagy properly. As you are fasting, most likely to lose weight, you should also be aware of the fact that if you only sleep for a limited amount of time, it means that you are more likely to be more hungry. This issue is that your levels of leptin are falling. This is going to cause an increase in your appetite because leptin is an appetite hormone. When you think about this, look at it this way. You are a student in this example and its finals week. You should be asleep, so you have a clear mind, but you are nervous and panicked (which is understandable), and you are pulling an all-nighter to study. So you have kept yourself up now all night, and you're not sleeping. Your stomach is rumbling, and you can't focus, so you eat. In most cases, this causes people to binge on junk food. Instead, you should let yourself get healthy sleep, so your mind is focused and more alert. Also, you let your body have the chance to heal itself.

Humans are said to spend about a third of their entire life sleeping, and this obviously differs between the age of the human or their health conditions. Some people sleep much more than others, and there are many people who sleep less, but as a person spends a third of their life sleeping, knowing how to properly trigger autophagy the way that your body needs to is going to help you. It is not uncommon for people to find it difficult to get going in the morning or even to rise from their bed. Unsurprisingly, this is an actual condition. This is different from waking up on Monday morning and feeling tired and listless. This is most likely due to the fact that your sleep schedule is altered on the weekends, and you are trying to get yourself back on your normal sleep schedule. The condition of not wanting to get out of bed is different, and studies are being done as to why this is and how to find coping solutions.

As you are trying to trigger your autophagy so you can start the process, you really want to make sure that you're having a restful sleep. When you wake up the next morning, you will find time to do some exercise at some part of your day because that is a trigger for autophagy as well. Sleep deprivation is actually something that can kill you more quickly than food deprivation (at least according to recent findings), which is why you really need to make sure that you get a proper amount of sleep because neither of these issues is good for you. There have been deaths reported from not sleeping, but the most famous case is perhaps the story of someone who died after staying up for eleven days straight. Your body needs the sleep to heal, so don't take this for granted, and make sure you are taking the time to sleep.

If sleep deprivation is going to possibly be fatal to you, then you'll obviously need to make sure that you're getting the proper amount of sleep. Find the balance for yourself, and remember that most people need between seven or nine hours. Once you find your balance and are making sure that you achieve this every night, you will begin to see a marked difference in your health and body. Your pain threshold is also reduced by sleep deprivation, so if you're not letting yourself get the proper amount of sleep each night, then your pain tolerance becomes much lower than it normally is. Studies have shown that falling asleep at night should only take you about a quarter of an hour or less ideally, but for many people, it takes longer because they need to power down their computers, or they're still on their phones. Another reason that sleep can evade them is if they have worries that they need to forget about but can't because they are plaguing their mind. Once you can power down and calm your mind, you may find that sleeping is much easier. This is why we've included the tips above so that you'll get a proper amount of sleep for your body and make sure that you are regaining your health.

Going without sleep is also more likely to make you hungry, and this makes you eat more, but there are other downsides to getting less sleep than required. For one, it is believed by certain studies that if you're awake for sixteen hours straight, it can cause a decrease in your performance that it becomes seriously noticeable. For instance, it is believed that staying awake for this long will decrease your performance as much as if your blood alcohol level were 0.5%. It should be noted here that the legal limit is 0.8%. That's really something to consider for people who find themselves doing this often because you are impairing your ability to function properly, but without knowing it, you could also be putting others in danger. Instead of letting this happen, make sure you get enough sleep and that you are taking care of yourself.

We've also mentioned in the earlier chapters that exercise can help sleep, as well. Regular exercise improves your sleep patterns, but exercising sporadically right before bed can actually keep you up. This is a shock for most people because they believe that if they exercise right before they go to bed, it will actually make them tired. However, this isn't true, and because of it, you can actually find yourself tossing or turning for a while before you are actually able to wind down and calm yourself into a relaxed state.

If you are able to fall asleep in less than five minutes, the chances are that you are seriously sleep-deprived (although, you could just be missing sleep less seriously or you are suffering from a sleep disorder). Sleep disorders are a serious issue, so if you're trying to learn how to trigger autophagy, this would be something to look into. Make sure that you are trying to get it under control so that you can sleep healthily without the disorder in the future or at least have it better managed.

Realistically, it should take a person between ten and twenty minutes to fall asleep. Women, according to recent studies, may actually need more sleep than men, and they also may suffer more when they don't get it. This is a subject of much debate and study, and as such, it is believed, at present, that women may suffer more mentally and physically if they are not able to get enough sleep. This could be due to the fact that women are said to be more multitasking than men. Because it is believed that women are bigger multitaskers, it is also believed that women may actually use more of their brain's functions than men do.

REM sleep maintains many different functions in both your brain and body. Autophagy maintains your neuronal axonal transport and functions as well. Rapid eye movement, which is known as REM sleep, is a unique psychological process that expressed in mammals. It also has effects on the different parts of your body and your brain.

Autophagy abnormalities can also be responsible for neuronal dysfunction, which can lead to death, and it can lead to different issues in your brain. Using different tactics and knowing helpful information is going to help you sleep better and understand how it's connected with autophagy. Studies (independent studies that need more research) have shown that dysfunction with autophagy is associated with diseases that are both chronic and acute in the neurodegenerative sense, and these are also related with losing sleep in the REM factor, which causes a heap of issues on its own. The best thing that you can do for your body and your health, especially if you're attempting autophagy, is to make sure that you're getting the proper amount of sleep, or it will cause further damage to your health.

Chapter 12: Supplementation and Integration

When you fast, there is the question of whether or not you should take food supplements or other useful supplements. Studies show that this depends on the situation. You have to think of the method of fast that you're using, the supplements involved, and individual needs. It's also important to check with your doctor.

Pregnant women should also never use any supplements without their doctor's permission because it could cause damage to the unborn child, as well as yourself.

As a good rule of thumb, if you already rely on a supplement for your normal routine, then you should continue using them on a fast. A good example is if you are someone who has a B12 deficiency, you should be aware that during the course of the fast, you may need a supplement to keep your levels in check and at a good level.

The type of fasting you choose informs you of the degree of how you restrict your calories. Since limiting the calories means sacrificing nutrients, many people turn to supplements. Usual concerns include whether or not they should take one in the first place and to what extent. Also, should one continue to use them if they already do and if there are recommended ones that they should use during a fast.

Also, is it possible to take short-term use supplements? One needs to realize that the answer to that question depends on other factors that need to be taken into account.

Studies go back and forth, but some believe it is not necessary to take vitamins while fasting, while others encourage it. The ones who don't believe that this is a necessary process believe that humans should be equipped for handling a reduced food supply. This changes, of course, if you already have an illness or other issues that are causing you problems. Others are concerned about their fitness levels being compromised, so they wonder if they should take protein powder to help their muscle atrophy. Studies show that supplements usually don't help very much during fasting and may be counterproductive. It is believed by others (such as from a naturopathic perspective) that a certain degree of degradation of protein through fasting serves some purpose, such as relieving inflammation.

Inflammation is believed to be a result of an overabundance of protein that is found in some diets.

If you lose muscle during a fast, it can be regained after, so you shouldn't worry about this too much. Another thing to note is that if you are ingesting amino acid supplements or protein powders, it stimulates insulin secretion. This is going to change your metabolism, and it can result in different fasting results. Intermittent fasting promotes food intake during window hours; studies believe that you should be able to preserve a baseline that is healthy concerning substances in your body.

A person also cannot go without vitamins, such as vitamin B12, D, zinc, and magnesium, based on specific health circumstances. In addition to this, it is said that if you suffer from a severe illness, then you should be consulting with the experts so that you are aware of what you need and how to take care of your body properly.

Chia seeds and flaxseeds are believed to activate the bowels and intestines during a. This is particularly believed to be true if the intestinal activity is slowed during a fast. The seeds should help stimulate your intestinal activity. In a fast, your digestion and bowel movements should remain regular, and as such, these seeds can help. When you take digestive foods (like the flaxseed) with a healthy amount of water, they swell in the intestines. This stimulates peristalsis for you. It is worth noting that flaxseeds should not be mortared or ground, as you will benefit from the effect and not the content.

If your doctor gives you permission, you can look into chlorophyll drops. These are supposed to be a great source for removing toxins while providing your body with the ability to prevent odors that can arise from a fast. As a side note, the drops do not affect your insulin levels or blood sugar.

If you have gotten permission to use supplements on a fast, then you should be aware of the following things. You need to make sure that your supplements are affecting your insulin and glucose levels. If they are, you need to stop and speak with your doctor right away. You should also pay attention to food supplements, as the sugar that you get from them can be found in fruits. Food supplements also cause diarrhea, nausea, and stomach aches.

Another thing that you need to be aware of is whether or not the supplements are fat-soluble. Your body would not receive a benefit from a supplement that includes little or no fat during a fast. Instead, you can eat fat-soluble food additions, along with foods that will give you the necessary vitamins, such as A, K, E, and D.

You will also need to be aware of the amount of medication that you take. The reason for this is that your medications are going to interact with your supplements, and it can harm you. In many cases, your doctor will express that you should not be taking supplements at all when you take medication.

Whether or not you should take supplements on a fast is a personal decision between you and your doctor. This is because there are many health issues that you could have, and taking a supplement could exacerbate it. In other circumstances, if you have an underlying health issue that you don't know about, using supplements on a fast could bring this issue to the forefront. If your doctor said it is alright to use supplements, then you should be alright to use these as long as you make sure to listen to both the doctor and your body. If you feel any discomfort or side effects, you should stop immediately because this is your body telling you something.

Conclusion

Autophagy is a concept that has gained popularity in recent years, and many studies have been conducted on the subject. In this book, we have covered a plethora of topics that you understand much better now and allow you to use to your benefit. We explained what metabolic autophagy is and how you can use this to your advantage. We also explained the cons of this, as well as the negatives that have been studied about the topic. It's important to know what you are getting into, and the best way is to get as much information as possible so that you understand what it does.

Fasting is a big trend right now, and this is something that we went over as well. There are many people who have said it's a good thing to do; however, these people need to realize that they are not medically trained, and they could be giving you bad information, leading you into something that might not be good for you. This is the reason that you need to seek advice from a professional or doctor because they know what would be best for your health.

In this book, we have relayed what intermittent fasting is and how it has been a very popularized diet. We've also covered why this type of fasting is different from regular fasting. It is something that hundreds of people attempt to try, but we explained that you need to do this safely so that you can stay healthy. We also explained how it's going to relate to what you're trying to do with your body and health, along with how the food you eat affects what you are feeling and how you're doing. One of the things that we have made sure to explain is the difference between anabolic and catabolic and how they are intricately linked with each other. This is going to help you when you're trying to adopt this for yourself. There are certain things that anabolic does for you that catabolism cannot and vice versa, and there are different foods for each process.

In addition, we have explained the importance of not fasting and the dangers of doing so when you're not in optimal health. There are specific conditions when fasting should not be attempted, such as in the event of disease. Infants and children should not fast at all because it's dangerous and can be fatal. We have also included the types of meals that you should be eating, and we'll explain the science behind it so that you have an accurate look of what you should ingest and how it affects your metabolic rate.

There are many different foods that you can eat when you're trying to understand your anabolism and catabolism. Because we understand that getting healthier can be really expensive, we have given you a thorough list of food that you can eat and which are affordable. Affordability tends to be on the list of reasons that you don't undergo this diet, but we've provided you with great examples of food that is available anywhere. These food items are good for your body. Many of the foods that we have listed can be prepared in such a way that will cut the cost but not the nutrients. Knowing the science behind this is important because it allows you to understand how this is going to affect your body and how it will affect your mind. Food affects both, and knowing this and understanding this will make you stronger because you will see and feel the effects.

You may not realize it, but autophagy affects how you sleep as well. This has to do with your circadian rhythm. It can be hard to stay on autophagy when you do not sleep well, so we provided tips for having the best sleep.

Being able to have a healthy sleep is going to heal your body, as well as your mind, and this is particularly true if you are getting a full night's sleep because it's going to have great repairing properties for you. It will also make you a much healthier person.

The tips that we've given you here should help you to understand autophagy and how to utilize these skills safely and healthily while using them to your benefit.

Made in the USA
Coppell, TX
06 February 2025

45538417R00095